P9-APH-930

ACQUIRED NEUROGENIC DISORDERS

REMEDIATION OF COMMUNICATION DISORDERS SERIES
Frederick N. Martin, Series Editor

STUTTERING

——————————————————————————— *Edward G. Conture*

HEARING IMPAIRMENTS IN YOUNG CHILDREN

——————————————————————————— *Arthur Boothroyd*

HARD OF HEARING CHILDREN IN REGULAR SCHOOLS

Mark Ross with Diane Brackett
——————————————————————— *and Antonia Maxon*

HEARING-HANDICAPPED ADULTS

——————————————————————————— *Thomas G. Giolas*

ACQUIRED NEUROGENIC DISORDERS

——————————————————————————— *Thomas P. Marquardt*

LANGUAGE DISORDERS IN PRESCHOOL CHILDREN

——————————————————————————— *Patricia R. Cole*

LANGUAGE DISORDERS IN SCHOOL AGE CHILDREN

——————————————————————————— *Mary Lovey Wood*

Forthcoming

ARTICULATION DISORDERS

——————————————————————————— *Ronald K. Sommers*

CEREBRAL PALSY

——————————————————————————— *James C. Hardy*

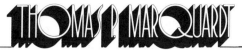

Thomas P. Marquardt

The University of Texas at Austin

ACQUIRED NEUROGENIC DISORDERS

Prentice-Hall, Inc., Englewood Cliffs, New Jersey 07632

Library of Congress Cataloging in Publication Data

Marquardt, Thomas P.
   Acquired neurogenic disorders.

   (Remediation of communication disorders series)
   Bibliography: p.
   Includes index.
   1. Speech, Disorders of. 2. Language disorders.
3. Brain damage—Complications and sequelae. 4. Com-
municative disorders. I. Title. II. Series: Remediation
of communication disorders. [DNLM. 1. Brain damage,
Chronic—Complications. 2. Speech disorders—Etiology.
WL 340 M357a]
RC423.M285   616.85'52   81-21081
ISBN 0-13-003814-8   AACR2

TO BARB AND TIMMY

Printed in the United States of America

10 9 8 7 6 5 4 3 2 1

Editorial/production supervision by Virginia Cavanagh Neri
Interior design by Maureen Olsen
Cover design by Maureen Olsen
Manufacturing buyer: Edmund W. Leone

ISBN 0-13-003814-8

Prentice-Hall International, Inc., *London*
Prentice-Hall of Australia Pty. Limited, *Sydney*
Prentice-Hall of Canada, Ltd., *Toronto*
Prentice-Hall of India Private Limited, *New Delhi*
Prentice-Hall of Japan, Inc., *Tokyo*
Prentice-Hall of Southeast Asia Pte. Ltd., *Singapore*
Whitehall Books Limited, *Wellington, New Zealand*

#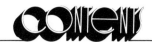

The disorders 1

The evaluation 22

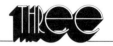

Prognosis 66

Therapy form and content 105

The rehabilitation process   156

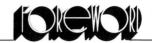

With the information explosion of recent years there has been a proliferation of knowledge in the areas of scientific and social inquiry. The speciality of communicative disorders has been no exception. While two decades ago a single textbook or "handbook" might have sufficed to provide the aspiring or practicing clinician with enlightenment on an array of communication handicaps, this is no longer possible—hence the decision to prepare a series of single-author texts.

As the title implies, the emphasis of this series, *Remediation of Communication Disorders,* is on therapy and treatment. The authors of each book were asked to provide information relative to anatomical and physiological aspects of each disorder, as well as pathology, etiology, and diagnosis to the extent that an understanding of these factors bears on management procedures. In such relatively short books this was quite a challenge: to offer guidance without writing a "cookbook"; to be selective without being parochial; to offer theory without losing sight of practice. To this challenge the series' authors have risen magnificently.

Thomas Marquardt has extensive clinical experience in the rehabilitation of patients with neurogenic communication disorders. He has served as a Veterans Administration trainee, was founder and coordinator of the University of Tennessee Neuropathology Services Program, and currently consults for several state and federal agencies, in addition to working with patients at The University of Texas Speech and Hearing Center. A member of that rare breed of researcher-clinicians, Dr. Marquardt is a superb teacher, a talent that is revealed in this book.

FREDERICK N. MARTIN
Series Editor

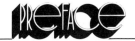

PREFACE

Acquired Neurogenic Disorders is intended to serve as a basic resource for speech/language pathologists in practice and for students in training. Physical and occupational therapists, neuropsychologists, nurses, and physicians also should find it of value in their work. The scope is comprehensive in that the major communicative disorders due to brain damage are reviewed. However, the focus clearly is on clinical procedures. An effort has been made to avoid biases in terminology and to provide as broad a review as possible of available clinical procedures. The first four chapters deal with specific topics: description, evaluation, prognosis, and treatment methods. The final chapter considers the longitudinal processes involved in treatment of the patient from referral to discharge and includes discussion of direct treatment, counseling, and structuring the communicative environment for the patient.

○ ACKNOWLEDGMENTS

This text could not have been completed without the help of patients, students, and collegues. I would especially like to acknowledge the aid of Jean Herzog in the preparation of artwork and for comments regarding content; Alice Richardson, Rick Bollinger, and John Tonkovich for materials and suggested revisions; Cindra O'Leary and Manda Van Geem for manuscript preparation; and Fred Martin, Series Editor, for commments regarding organization and style.

THOMAS P. MARQUARDT

ACQUIRED NEUROGENIC DISORDERS

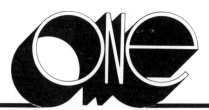

The disorders

○ INTRODUCTION

Neurologically impaired adults display an array of speech and language deficits, ranging from readily observable motor speech disorders to more subtle impairments of language and cognition. Rehabilitating these patients involves a series of overlapping tasks: identifying the problem, determining a prognosis, implementing a treatment program, and evaluating progress. Each stage of this process requires that a balance be struck between what is known and what is hypothesized about the patient and the disorder. Russell Brain, the eminent British neurologist, succinctly described this balance when he observed that "progress . . . depends upon the ability to ride with a foot on each of two horses, one named Fact and one named Hypothesis, and the problem always to keep them running level" (1966, p. 566). The primary goal of this book is to provide a balanced account of rehabilitation facts and hypotheses that can be used to help brain-injured adults recover their communication skills. To accomplish this purpose, both a rationale for treatment and specific procedures will be discussed.

The communication disorders to be considered are termed *acquired* and *neurogenic*. Acquired indicates that the communication deficits occurred after speech and language was developed. Neurogenic specifies that the disorders are due to damage to the nervous system.

There is no universal acceptance of diagnostic labels to describe neurogenic disorders. Perhaps the only agreement is that there is no agreement. Historically, investigators devised terms, using symptom complexes to localize speech and language functions of the brain. *Nosology* reflected the neural function inferred (e.g., *motor, sensory*) or the investigator's surname (e.g. *Broca, Wernicke*). Investigators also used descriptive labels based on the primary characteristics of the disorder (e.g., *jargon, agrammatism, phonetic disintegration*) and interchangeably used terms such as *dysarthria* for relatively distinctive neuromuscular and nonneuromuscularly based deficits. An example may illustrate the large number of terms for a symptom complex: A disorder due to anterior dominant hemisphere brain damage with a primary deficit in the ability to program articulatory movements has been variously labeled *motor aphasia, Broca's aphasia, primarily expressive aphasia, phonetic disintegration, cortical dysarthria,* and *apraxia of speech.*

2

Reviewing all the terminology and classification systems for communication problems due to brain damage would serve little purpose. The first task here will be to describe three frequently encountered communication problems associated with nervous system pathology: *aphasia, apraxia,* and *dysarthria.* Aphasia is a language disorder caused by injury to the dominant hemisphere responsible for processing the language code. Apraxia is a motor speech disorder resulting from damage to neural circuits of the dominant hemisphere responsible for programming speech movements. Dysarthria is a neuromuscular speech disorder characterized by weakness, paralysis, and/or incoordination.

These three terms and the parameters of the disorders they label are not universally agreed upon. They will be used because they are convenient, not because they are right or wrong; numerous therapy approaches are directed at disorders for which these terms serve as descriptive abbreviations. The behavioral variations, not the labels, are of real importance.

Aphasia, apraxia, and dysarthria are not mutually exclusive deficits, and each or all may be demonstrated by a brain-damaged patient. In fact, no one symptom is unique to a given diagnostic category. These disorders are frequently complicated by memory, orientation, judgment, cognition, visuospatial, and visuomotor deficits. Disorders of this type will be examined secondarily and only because knowledge of their characteristics is necessary to describe the entire communication impairment of the patient and because speech-language pathologists are increasingly called upon to evaluate and treat patients with nondominant hemisphere and bihemisphere lesions who demonstrate these deficits.

Chapter One will include an elementary neurological framework, some limited information on etiology, and a review of the primary characteristics of the disorder. Additional definition of these topics will evolve from the discussion of appraisal and diagnosis.

Description of communication problems is aided by test instruments used to quantify characteristics of the disorder. Whether the tests are of language, intellect, memory, cognition, or motor speech, their purpose is to provide the empirical data base for differential diagnosis—the process of labeling the disorder. This descriptive process is important because it isolates the communication problems to be addressed and because different disorders require different therapeutic techniques. Chapter Two will consider appraisal and diagnosis of neurogenic disorders. The emphasis will be on test instruments of appraisal with more limited discussion of differential diagnosis. Diagnostic decision making will be considered more fully later.

Not all patients with nervous system injury will benefit from direct treatment of their communication disorder, and it is important to determine the prognosis for recovery as soon as possible in the rehabilitation process. *Prognosis* is a prediction of treatment outcome based on factual indicants of the patient's condition. Prognostic indicators include variables such as location and size of the lesion, presence or absence of sensory and motor impairments, age, intellectual ability, educational level, and emotional and psychological adjustment of the patient. In few other communication disorders has prognosis been as consistently neglected under the assumption that some treatment is better than no treatment and that any progress is sufficient to justify the therapeutic effort. Judicious use of prognostic indicators is of significant value in determining the procedures to be used and in devising reasonable expectations for the patient. Chapter Three will deal with predictors of treatment outcome, the efficacy of treatment, and aspects of spontaneous recovery.

Therapy approaches have both form and content. Therapy forms for neurogenic disorders are a study in contrasts, ranging from regimented programmed instruction based on operant principles to unstructured conversation used to maximize residual communicative abilities. Therapy content is determined by the disorder to be treated and the needs of the patient. Chapter Four will deal with therapy rationales and procedures.

Finally, the processes of rehabilitation from referral of the patient to termination of treatment will be considered. While the first four chapters are relatively self-contained, Chapter Five describes the multifaceted and interconnected roles of the clinician as diagnostician, prognosticator, treatment provider, and counselor.

This brief introduction has emphasized that rehabilitation of acquired neurogenic communication disorders is a dynamic process involving a continual reassessment of the diagnosis, prognosis, and treatment program. The following description and evaluation of rehabilitation facts and hypotheses should enhance the clinician's delivery of services to these communicatively handicapped patients.

○ NEUROLOGICAL BASES OF ACQUIRED DISORDERS

introduction

An elementary knowledge of functional neuroanatomy, etiologies of brain damage, and characteristics of acquired disorders are required to understand the rehabilitation process. In the following sections, a functional topography of the nervous system is developed, etiologies of brain damage are examined, and the characteristics of acquired disorders are described.

the nervous system

The nervous system can be divided into two parts: central and peripheral. The *central nervous system* includes the *cerebrum* divided into two structurally similar but functionally dissimilar hemispheres with *frontal, tem-*

poral, parietal, and *occipital* lobes; the *brain stem* including the *midbrain, pons,* and *medulla;* the *cerebellum* with anatomically but not functionally identical halves; and the *spinal cord* (Figure 1–1). The central nervous system is encased in bone, surrounded by cerebrospinal fluid and covered by meningeal layers. The *peripheral nervous system* is composed of nerves that extend from the central nervous system (Figure 1–2). The *cranial nerves* primarily subserve the head and neck, and the *spinal nerves* innervate the rest of the body. Within the nervous system are pathways that convey sensory information from the periphery to the central nervous system and motor pathways that carry impulses from the neuroaxis to the muscles and glands which serve as effector organs. Each level of the central nervous system has interconnections between the two sides, between sensory and motor systems, and between higher and lower structures. The three components of the system to be examined are the dominant hemisphere for speech and language, the nondominant hemisphere, and the motor systems.

The Dominant Hemisphere. Both hemispheres of the brain are capable of establishing verbal processes at birth, but as the organism matures, a genetically predetermined displacement assigns verbal functions to the left hemisphere and visuospatial and other nonverbal functions to the

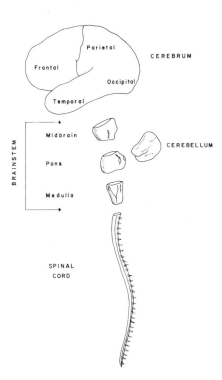

FIGURE 1–1 Subdivisions of the Central Nervous System

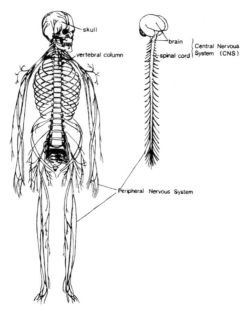

FIGURE 1–2 Central and Peripheral nervous systems. From G. Dunkerley, *A Basic Atlas of the Human Nervous System.* Philadelphia: F. A. Davis Co., 1975. Reprinted by permission.

right hemisphere. The dominance is functional, not anatomical, although the left and right hemispheres have some structural differences (LeMay and Geschwind, 1978). Consequently almost all right-handed and most left-handed individuals have left hemisphere dominance for speech and language activities.

Although the left hemisphere is generally accepted as having a preponderant role in verbal functioning, the nature of the relationship between cortical areas and function is less agreed upon. Much of the early work on localization of function was based on postmortem data. Patients with disorders due to nervous system impairment were evaluated, and their brains were examined after death in an effort to correlate behavioral characteristics with specific sites of lesion. More recently cortical mapping by electrostimulation (Penfield and Roberts, 1959), regional blood flow studies (Ingvar, 1976; Lassen, Ingvar, and Skinhoj, 1978), and large sample missile wound investigations (Luria, 1970; Russell & Espir, 1961) have been primary sources of new data. Surprisingly investigators utilizing comparable subject populations and similar behavioral measures have not reached agreement on the specificity of cortical representation of function. At one end of the spectrum are those researchers such as Geschwind (1965) who suggest that constellations of language impairments can be accounted for on the basis of circumscribed lesions. At the other end of the spectrum are investigators such as Bay (1967) and Schuell, Jenkins, and Jimenez-Pabon (1964) who suggest that language impairments have limited, if any, localizing value.

With such incompatible conceptualizations of functional specialization of the dominant hemisphere, how is it possible to generate a principled account of topographic representation which can serve as scaffolding for descriptions of speech and language deficits? A place to begin is by noting the dynamic characteristics of cortical activity. The brain is continuously active. The level of excitation and extent of heightened activity is determined by the processing demands of the task (Lassen et al., 1978). Additionally as Lenneberg (1975) has noted, the brain has such a complex anatomical connectivity that no part is isolated functionally from all other parts. A lesion will not destroy a particular cortical area and its corresponding function but will deform the normal pattern of interaction of a whole network of activities. Damage to the dominant hemisphere, according to Lenneberg, will produce disturbances on a variety of tasks and will usually affect some more than others, depending on the site and extent of lesion.

A topographic representation of the brain requires that the dynamic aspects of its processing activity be considered. Localizing cortical representation and specifying locations of damage that cause altered activity are two different tasks; an attempt will be made, however, to define a middle ground between a strict localization of function viewpoint and the theories that suggest relative equipotentiality of the cortex.

A lateral view of the left hemisphere is presented in Figure 1–3. Structural landmarks are identified for each of the lobes. It is generally agreed that the occipital lobe mediates vision, the postcentral gyrus of the parietal lobe mediates muscle and skin senses, the precentral gyrus of the frontal lobe subserves motor activities and portions of the temporal gyri mediate audition. Large areas of the left hemisphere do not perform specific sensory or motor functions but are given over to detailed sensory analysis, motor

FIGURE 1–3 Lateral Aspect of the Left Cerebral Hemisphere

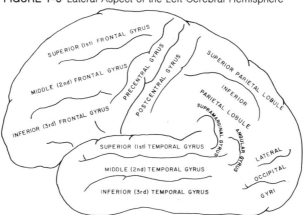

planning, and other mental activities. Regions that give rise to unique functions extend from the inferior posterior frontal lobe to the superior posterior temporal lobe. Within this region are primary cortical representation areas for verbal processes.

Efforts to set absolute boundaries on the language representation cortical areas have been at the heart of most localization controversies. Based upon probability distribution hypotheses proposed by Bogen and Bogen (1977) and cortical excitation propositions suggested by Lenneberg (1975), specifying two parameters appears to be minimally sufficient to designate the verbal processing regions of the dominant hemisphere. First, what are the regions that are primarily responsible for subserving these skills? Secondly, what is the relationship between these areas and verbal functions?

Many types of data might be used to specify the cortical regions responsible for verbal processing. For convenience, evidence from missile wounds will serve as a starting point. Figure 1–4 from Russell (1963) shows the area of the brain within which a small wound will cause language disturbances. Two aspects of Figure 1–4 are particularly noteworthy. First, the area includes the lowermost part of the third frontal gyrus (Broca's area) and postcentral gyrus, the supramarginal and angular gyri, the inferior parietal gyri, and the superior aspect of the temporal lobe (including Wernicke's area). Second, the figure shows that a very small probability exists that damage to the periphery of the hemisphere—the temporal, frontal, and occipital poles—will cause significant linguistic deficits.

Russell's figure is useful but insufficient because it implies an equal representational density within the area and little or no representation outside of it. This problem can be overcome by viewing the demarcated area as a region containing several centers with relatively greater responsibility for verbal processing and whose effect decreases with increasing distance, like a gravity field. The epicenters of high verbal functional density have been well established from cortical mapping, blood flow studies, and postmortem

FIGURE 1–4 Limits of the area of the brain within which a small wound will cause language deficits. From W. Russell, Some anatomical aspects of aphasia. *Lancet,* 1963, *1,* 1173-1177. Reprinted by permission.

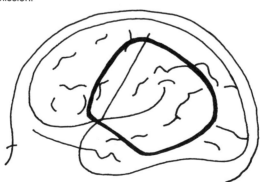

data. One primary center lies on the posterior portion of the third frontal gyrus (Broca's area) and the other on the first temporal gyrus (Wernicke's area). What has been established thus far, then, is an extensive verbal representational field with at least two centers.

The next consideration is the specific representation of functions within the field. There is little question that area and function are correlated. The real question is the specificity with which these functions are assigned to circumscribed areas. Given the anatomical connectivity of the brain and its constant activity, it is difficult to conceive of functions assigned to exact cortical locations like a mosaic. A more reasoned view is that specific language processes are represented over a fairly large area of the cortex with a great deal of overlap between functions. Consequently any given cortical area within the representational area for language could be viewed as a series of functional layers with the depth of the layer determined by the density of activity for a particular linguistic process. Knowing that anterior areas of the cortical regions for language are more responsible for expressive skills while posterior regions are more responsible for receptive skills, it would be argued that a lesion would cause multiple linguistic processing deficits with the severity of any given impairment dependent upon the site of lesion and the severity of the overall deficit defined by the extent of tissue loss relative to the representational centers.

This topographic view of cortical representation is supported by Figure 1–5 from Luria (1964) that shows the percentage of discrimination deficits in 800 patients with missile wounds to the left hemisphere. The discrimination deficits, according to Luria, are the primary defect of language comprehension disorders due to damage to the posterior speech (Wernicke's) area. The highest frequency of disorders arise from damage to this area, the second highest incidence is associated with more anterior damage, and only minimal or no deficits are apparent at the perimeter of the hemisphere.

In summary, the dominant hemisphere is responsible for processing linguistic elements. The cortical representation of these processes is not static and subject to an exact demarcation. Rather, language representation is in the form of functional gravity fields within which the representation of specific skills overlaps with that of other linguistic and symbolic abilities.

The foregoing description is greatly oversimplified and does not include important participation by the nondominant hemisphere and subcortical structures in verbal and cognitive processes. It does, however, bring into focus the idea that no disorder syndrome is independent from all others or can be because the neurological structures subserving verbal processing are united in a complex way.

The "Nondominant" Hemisphere. The term *nondominant* refers to the half of the brain not primarily responsible for language. It does not suggest that the hemisphere is inactive during speech and language activities. It is a participant, although not the preponderant functional half of the

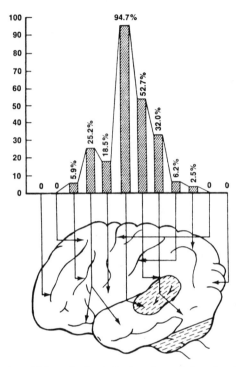

FIGURE 1-5 The number of failures in discrimination of correlative phonemes in different lesions (based on 800 observations of missile wounds of the left hemisphere). From A. R. Luria, Factors and forms of aphasia. In A. DeReuck, and M. O'Connor, (Eds.), *Disorders of language*. London: The Ciba Foundation, 1964, p. 148. Reprinted by permission.

brain involved in linguistic processing (Kinsbourne, 1975; Lassen et al., 1978).

The nondominant hemisphere is structurally similar (LeMay and Geschwind, 1978) to the dominant but demonstrates a number of functions that are unique. Reviews of right hemisphere functioning (Gates and Bradshaw, 1977; Joynt and Goldstein, 1975; Krashen, 1976) suggest that this hemisphere plays a significant role in spatial perception, body image, visual perception, and constructional abilities. It also has functions relative to musical abilities and elementary speech, including recognition and use of musical tones and patterns, verbal processing of some words, and overlearned phrases. A more detailed consideration of right hemisphere participation in language will be present in the discussion of spontaneous recovery following brain damage.

Motor Systems Arising from the cortex are two interconnected motor systems. The *pyramidal* tract is the motor system of voluntary control and has two components. The corticobulbar portion is made up of upper motor neurons that provide innervation bilaterally to the motor nuclei of the cranial nerves in the brain stem. The corticospinal fibers provide innervation primarily to contralateral motor nuclei of the spinal nerves after arising from the cortex and following a major decussation of approximately 80 percent of the fibers at the base of the medulla. The pyramidal tract provides a direct pathway from the cortex to muscles by means of upper motor neurons (*corticobulbar* and *corticospinal* pathways) to lower motor neurons (cranial and spinal nerves) to muscles. The major function of the tract is to produce rapid phasic movements.

The phylogenetically older *extrapyramidal* tract includes nonreflex motor pathways not included in the pyramidal tract. The tract arises primarily from the frontal lobes, but its major structures are subcortical nuclei, including the *basal ganglia (caudate, putamen, globus pallidus)* and two other paired structures of the upper brainstem *(subthalamus, red nucleus)*. The nuclei have three types of connecting fibers including interconnections with higher motor systems, intrinsic connections among the nuclei, and efferent projections to lower motor neurons (Darley, Aronson, and Brown, 1975). The extrapyramidal system has a major role in sustained tonic aspects of movement. Its activity is primarily inhibitory.

The role of the *cerebellum* is to coordinate the timing of activity in various muscle groups for locomotion, posture, and volitional motor acts. This function is accomplished by modulation of motor activity arising elsewhere in the nervous system based upon information received from the cerebral cortex and sensory receptors.

Netsell (1975) has provided an elementary motor control model (Figure 1–6) that facilitates description of the motor system because of its emphasis on function rather than structure and which is paraphrased here. Vertically, the model shows a division of the system into central nervous system, peripheral nervous system, and mechanical system.

The mechanical system (MS) is represented by the responses of the system designated as muscle contractions and movements of the speech production structures. The movement is determined by the muscular and nonmuscular forces operating on that part. Immediately above the mechanical system is the peripheral nervous system (PNS). The PNS includes the spinal and cranial nerves and is represented by motoneurons (MNs) in the PNS nuclei. The PNS and the muscles innervated by it are identified as the effectors of the responses (muscle contractions and movements). They operate as passive elements in the total system and respond to the central nervous system (CNS) controls.

The central nervous system is represented in the diagram by two control systems into which are input three control variables. The controller systems are identified as the movement control system (MCS) and the postural control system (PCS). The control variables are strength (S), timing (Ti) and tone (To). The strength variable is determined by the firing rate of upper motor neurons and the number of neurons participating. Timing refers to

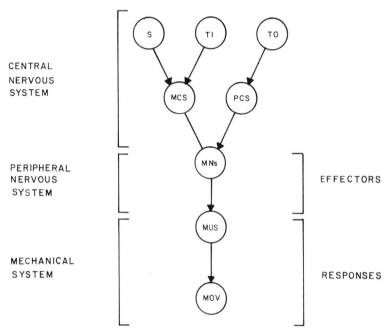

FIGURE 1–6 Model of Speech Motor Control. Adapted from R. Netsell, *Kinesiology studies of the dysarthrias.* Madison: University of Wisconsin, 1975. Reprinted by permission.

the control variable that regulates the onset, duration, and offset of the strength variable. Implicit in this concept of timing is reciprocity; some muscles are actively inhibited while the Central Motor Neurons (CMNs) controlling the prime movers are excited. The organism learns to pattern these variables of strength and timing to drive the speech production musculature. The tone input is the amount of background tension upon which the MCS operates to direct specific patterns of contractions for speech movements.

Netsell's model is useful for describing neuromuscular speech disorders because it allows quantitative as well as qualitative views of the underlying altered muscle function. That is, the dysarthrias can be considered in terms of abnormal strength, timing, and tone.

○ ETIOLOGIES OF NERVOUS SYSTEM DYSFUNCTION

Nervous system impairment results from cerebrovascular, traumatic, neoplastic, infectious, or degenerative changes; etiologies that are not mutually exclusive. They will be briefly described here. The time course of nervous system physiological events subsequent to damage will be examined in more detail later.

The major cerebrovascular sources of brain damage occur against the backdrop of plaquelike material build up in arterial walls. *Thrombosis* is the terminal occlusion of an artery following gradual stenosis. An *embolus* is a moving clot of thrombotic tissue, air, or fat dislodged from another part of the body which occludes the blood vessel. The effect of thrombotic or embolic occlusion is to restrict the flow of oxygen-rich blood to brain tissue. The brain cells, cut off from oxygen, suffer from ischemia and die. *Hemorrhage* is a bleeding from a vessel into surrounding brain tissue which prevents nutrients and oxygen from reaching brain cells. In the majority of cases, the hemorrhage results from a ruptured arteriosclerotic artery and is followed by replacement of blood and brain tissue with connective tissue, glia, and new blood vessels (Chusid, 1970). When associated with atherosclerosis, hemorrhages frequently are preceded by an *aneurysm*—a dilation of the vessel due to a defective arterial wall. The effect of the hemorrhagic mass is to compress surrounding neural structures.

A second major source of nervous system damage is *trauma.* The useful distinctions for describing these lesions are based on the nature of the skull injury. Closed-head injuries are caused by absorption of mechanical energy by the head without penetration of the skull. They vary in severity from indentation caused by light blows to simple fractures caused when greater force is applied. The effect of the cranial blow is to produce contusions. Coup lesions are found at the point of impact due to direct trauma; contracoup lesions at the other end of the brain are due to displacement of the brain against the inner surface of the skull. With complex fracturing and depression of the skull, the underlying meningeal layers and brain are lacerated at the point of impact. *Penetrating wounds,* caused most often from gunshot, produce brain damage in the path of entry; this term is reserved for lesions produced by missiles that do not leave the skull cavity. *Perforating wounds* are produced by missiles that pass through the skull. Hemorrhages (e.g., subdural, subarachnoid, intracerebral) and direct tissue destruction are common findings subsequent to traumatic etiologies.

Neoplasms are abnormal growths within the brain or surrounding tissues. They arise from neuroglial cells and track between normal nerve cells without destroying them. The location of the tumor rather than its histology generally determine the deficits observed (Lewis, 1976). Increased intracranial pressure is produced not only by the space-occupying effect of the mass but also by a markedly altered circulatory pattern (Baptista, 1976), decreased blood flow, edema, structural displacement, and diffuse depression of function. Surgical resection of the abnormal mass destroys brain tissue.

Numerous etiological agents produce inflammatory or infectious lesions of the central nervous system. Most typically they are bacterial or viral microorganisms that invade by one of the following routes: (1) via the bloodstream, (2) by direct access from the environment, (3) from infected cavities adjacent to the cranium, or (4) along axons of motor and sensory neurons (Lewis, 1976). A virus is a microorganism that cannot proliferate outside of its host cell; bacteria, however, may exist within a host cell or extracellularly. *Meningitis* is an inflammation of the subarachnoid area; *encephalitis* is an inflammation of brain tissue. Recovery depends on the body's ability to restrict the infection. Brain abscesses are a complication of bacterial infection and consist of a walled-off cavity containing dead or dying white blood cells. These abscesses destroy tissue at the site and may produce increased intracranial pressure.

Finally, there are progressive degenerative nervous system changes and toxic and/or metabolic disturbances that affect neural function. Degeneration produces permanent diffuse and/or focal lesions; toxic and metabolic changes bring about reversible alterations in neural function or generate permanent structural defects insensitive to medical intervention.

○ NEUROGENIC COMMUNICATION DISORDERS: DEFINITION AND DESCRIPTION

Aphasia Cerebrovascular, traumatic, and brain abscess lesions to the language representation areas of the dominant hemisphere are primary causes of aphasia. Aphasia is a multimodality language impairment characterized by reduced ability to encode and decode linguistic units. Reading, writing, speaking, and comprehension abilities are involved. The linguistic impairment affects semantic, syntactic, lexical, and phonological aspects of the linguistic process. Patients will demonstrate an impoverished vocabulary, impaired ability to utilize more complex syntactic forms, and difficulty with more abstract and less frequently occurring words. They may also demonstrate phonemic errors, including paraphasias.

Aphasia has been viewed by some researchers as a unitary disorder. Schuell et al. (1964), for example, described five major and two minor syndromes in which aphasia was the major component. This classification suggests that aphasia is a singular disorder that may be complicated by sensory, motor, and dysarthric impairments. In contrast to this conceptualization, which Jakobsen (1964) termed a *unitarian heresy,* are classifications that suggest that constellations of disturbances can be reliably differentiated and that these syndromes can be localized to specific sites of lesion on the cortical representational area for language. For example, Goodglass and Kaplan (1972) described six major syndromes of aphasia and the corresponding cortical damage areas.

One important point regarding aphasia classification schemes must be emphasized. The care with which aphasic disturbances are described is more important than the schemes used to classify syndromes of impairment. A particular classification may be viewed through rose-colored glasses or a jaundiced eye depending upon the filter characteristics of our own biases, but the most important facet of the entire process for clinical practice is description.

Apraxia More than a hundred years ago Broca described an impairment in the production of speech caused by damage to the inferior posterior frontal lobe (Broca's area). The disorder subsequently has been named Broca's aphasia, apraxic dysarthria, motor aphasia, verbal aphasia and, more recently, apraxia of speech (Johns and La Pointe, 1976). Apraxia has been described by Darley et al. (1975) as impairment of neural circuitry responsible for programming articulatory movements and sequences of movements. Prosodic disturbances may be secondary characteristics of the disorder, perhaps in compensation for reduced ability to program movements. The disorder is considered to be independent of linguistic deficits and neuromuscular impairment although they may be seen as frequent concomitants of the syndrome.

The description provided by Darley et al. (1975) suggests that a cortical lesion may produce a nonlinguistic speech disorder due to a circumscribed lesion of the frontal lobe. This view of the deficit has not gone unchallenged (Martin, 1974). As noted earlier, the continual but varying excitability and anatomical connectivity of the cortex would preclude the development of a disorder independent of language deficits. Perhaps the disorder is best viewed as a syndrome in which the most prominent disturbances are in the programming of movements and in which linguistic deficits are evident but mild (Trost and Canter, 1974).

Several studies (Johns and Darley, 1970; La Pointe and Johns, 1975; Trost and Canter, 1974) have helped to specify the articulatory characteristics of apraxia. They have revealed that errors are not due to any specific muscle dysfunction, are primarily errors of complication than of simplification, and predominantly involve consonants rather than vowels. Apraxic speakers also make more errors on fricatives, affricatives, and consonant clusters than on other consonants. Since the disorder occurs frequently and therapy strategies have been developed specifically to deal with speech motor programming deficits, apraxia will receive considerable attention in the discussion of rehabilitation procedures.

Agnosia Another disorder due to dominant hemisphere brain damage is agnosia. Agnosia is a deficit in the ability to recognize stimuli through a sensory modality even though the pathway to the cortex is intact; that is, intact sensory input does not lead to recognition of the stimulus. Wepman (1951) suggested that agnosia is a nonlinguistic disorder. Since it seldom occurs in the absence of aphasia, discussion of its treatment will be combined with that of aphasia.

Deficits Associated with Right Brain Damage Cerebrovascular, traumatic, neoplastic, and infectious lesions of the nondominant hemisphere do not typically produce language disorders. They do, however, impair a number of nonlanguage functions often causing patients to be referred for evaluation and possible treatment. Joynt and Goldstein (1975), Brookshire (1978), and Leuteneggar (1975) have reviewed some of these impairments. They include spatial perception and body image disorders such as lack of awareness of, indifference to or denial of hemiparesis, inability to dress correctly, and topographical memory loss where the patient may become lost even in familiar environments. Visual perceptual disorders may also occur such as a reduced ability to identify familiar faces, left visual field problems, and difficult evaluating and integrating visual information. Visuospatial perception dysfunction also may cause constructional disabilities. The patient with right brain damage tends to be excessively verbose, demonstrates poor judgment, and has difficulty completing a task requiring a series of steps. He or she may also have problems in monitoring the passage of time and may frequently deny the existence of deficits.

Bihemispheric Syndromes—Confusion and Dementia Bilateral hemispheric symptomotology arises from structural changes in the brain or from interference with its normal activity. The syndromes may be divided into two types: *acute* and *chronic.*

Acute syndromes sometimes arise from a specific cause such as a traumatic or cerebrovascular based lesion. More often no structural damage to the brain has occurred, and the disturbance is due to a systemic dysfunction arising from cardiac failure, acute or chronic respiratory disease, surgical operation, dehydration and electrolytic disturbance, anemia, malignant disease, intoxication, or vitamin and nutritional disturbance (Kay, 1972). The syndrome usually is rapid in onset and is reversible in many cases. These disorders result from a process originating outside the nervous tissue which alters the environment of neurons without producing permanent structural changes (Foley, 1972).

Darley (1964) termed the type of the communicative impairment associated with acute bihemispheric involvement the *language of confusion.* He noted (Darley, 1964, 1975) that patients with this disorder have trouble recognizing, understanding and responding to the environment. They also have faulty short-term memory and mistaken reasoning, are disoriented in time and space, and have behavior which is less adaptive and appropriate than normal. Controlled investigations of the communicative disorders associated with acute syndromes are virtually nonexistent and limited primarily to clinical descriptions. A study by Halpern, Darley, and Brown (1973), however, shed some light on the most prominent features of the disorder. Comparing ten patients suffering from confusion with patients demonstrating aphasia, apraxia of speech, and dementia revealed that the confused patients were moderately impaired in arithmetic, reading comprehension, writing to dictation, and relevance. They were mildly impaired in communicative adequacy, auditory comprehension, syntax, naming, auditory retention, and fluency. With medical treatment and subsequent recovery, the confusional state of the patient would be expected to return to its premorbid level if the etiology does not produce significant loss of brain tissue.

In the chronic syndromes, the changes are usually widespread, severe, and progressive. This condition is typically called *dementia* and is due to a disease or group of diseases which cause cerebral atrophy and associated deterioration of mental processes. Dementia has multiple etiologies, all having in common a diffuse neuronal degeneration within the cerebral cortex. The degeneration takes the form of a loss of brain weight, dilation of the cerebral ventricles, appearance of senile plaques and neurofibrillary tangles, a widening of sulci, and a shrinking of the cortical ribbon (Berry, 1975; Brody, 1970).

The etiologies of the extensive cerebral deterioration may be divided into vascular and nonvascular. Vascular disorders arise from a progressive arteriosclerosis of the blood vessels or extensive multifocal infarcts. Nonvascular dementias include diseases of hereditary (e.g., Huntington's chorea), viral (e.g., Jakob-Creutzfeldt's disease), and metabolic (Wilson's disease) origin and those due to a progressive deterioration with loss of neurons for which a specific etiology has not been assigned (Alzheimer's disease) (Foley, 1972). On the whole, dementias, or chronic brain syndromes, are primarily associated with the aging process, but many of the structural changes in the brain associated with the disorder are also seen in nondemented elderly individuals (Tomlinson, Blessed, and Roth, 1970).

Miller (1977) has described the most salient features of dementia, such as a prominent impairment of memory, particularly for recent events; impoverished, concrete thinking which may lead to difficulty in coping with simple tasks; emotional alterations of which the most common is depression; and word-finding problems. Not all patients with dementia, however, will demonstrate this cluster of symptoms.

Darley (1964) has termed the disorder the *language of generalized intellectual deterioration.* As with the language of confusion, the disorder encompasses a complex of symptoms in addition to language deficits. Language functioning within this group has not been extensively explored. The available data suggests that word-finding and naming skills are disrupted (Barker and Lawson, 1968; Rochford, 1971), that reading comprehension and to a lesser extent auditory retention span are decreased (Halpern et al., 1973), and that language function may be isolated comparable to symtoms caused by widespread lesions of the dominant hemisphere (Whitaker, 1976). In an extensive review Ajuriaguerra and Tissot (1975) noted that the disintegration of language in dementia is the result of various types of disturbances, such as impoverishment of vocabulary, stereotyped repetition, inability to recall words, disordered syntax, and semantic and phonemic paraphasias. They proposed that the symptoms could not be reduced to a common denominator nor could the defects be attributed to a general intellectual decline or instrumental disturbances alone. They hypothesized that the language disorganization was due to a combination of breakdowns in various functions and processes of the cerebrum.

Two recent studies have provided information on language and communication in dementia. North and Ulatowska (1979) found that organic brain syndrome patients are prone to rely on perceptual, rather than conceptual, features to describe categories; to provide concrete, rather than abstract, responses; to make judgmental and evaluative comments; and to produce vague and undifferentiated responses on cognitive tasks. Richardson (1980) found that senile patients demonstrated more errors than their neurologically normal age-mates on seven error categories established from analysis of spontaneous and referential communication speech samples: misnaming, perseveration, uncertainty behaviors, fragmentation, referential unclarity, comprehension failure, and insensitivity to listener needs. All these categories fall within the domains of vocabulary, content, discourse, and use.

Dysarthria Dysarthrias are neuromuscular speech disorders arising from motor pathway damage at singular or multiple sites from the cortex to muscle. They may affect the entire speech production mechanism, including respiratory, phonatory, and articulatory processes, or be limited to more specific musculature. The type of dysarthria demonstrated will depend upon the site of lesion within the motor pathways.

A number of classification systems have been developed for the dysarthrias, including those based on the etiology of the disorder, the neuroanatomic site of lesion, or the disease entity which produced the disorder. The system proposed by Darley et al. (1975) will be used because it allows a partial meshing of the speech motor control model of Netsell with the perceptually based data of Darley et al.

Darley et al. (1975) described six types of dysarthria. *Flaccid* dysarthria was attributed to damage to the lower motor neuron. The effect of the damage would be, according to Netsell, a reduction or absence of muscle activity since the strength, timing, and tone inputs of the central nervous system are being played on an essentially nonfunctional lower motor neuron. The most prominent features of flaccid dysarthria are hypernasality, consonant imprecision, breathiness, and nasal emission.

Spastic dysarthria results from damage to the pyramidal tract, although components of the extrapyramidal system also have been implicated. Netsell suggested that the primary neuromuscular alteration for these patients is a reduction in the strength variable with apparently little alteration of tone or timing inputs. The major perceptual features of spastic dysarthria include consonant imprecision, monopitch, reduced stress, harsh voice quality, and monoloudness.

Lesions of the cerebellum produce *ataxic* dysarthria. The underlying neuromuscular basis of the disorder appears to be a reduction in tone (Kent and Netsell, 1975) which would produce weakness, although associated dysrhythmia may require other neuromuscular explanations. The primary perceptual characteristics of ataxic dysarthria are consonant imprecision, excess and equal stress, irregular articulatory breakdown, distorted vowels, and harsh voice quality.

Involvement of subcortical nuclei of the extrapyramidal tract result in *hypokinetic* or *hyperkinetic* dysarthrias. The primary example of *hypokinetic* dysarthria is Parkinson's disease. The suggested primary neuromuscular features of the disorder (Netsell, Daniel, and Celesia, 1975) are a balanced hypertonicity, reduced strength, and a disturbance in timing that may yield increased or decreased rate of movement. Key disturbed dimensions include monopitch, reduced stress, monoloudness, imprecise consonants, inappropriate silences, and short rushes of speech.

Hyperkinetic dysarthrias can be divided into those with fast involuntary movements and those with slow involuntary movements. Both involve a fluctuating hypertonicity in which random contractions occur in the muscles. A primary form of fast hyperkinetic dysarthria is chorea; an example of slow hyperkinetic dysarthria is dystonia. Hyperkinetic forms of dysarthira result primarily from damage to the extrapyramidal system. Characteristics of these disorders include consonant imprecision, prolonged intervals, slowed rate, distorted vowels, and irregular articulatory breakdowns. The disturbed dimensions for the two groups have a number of similar characteristics but are not identical.

Mixed dysarthrias result from damage to multiple points within the motor pathways. For example, multiple sclerosis may produce lesions of the spinal cord, brain stem, cerebellum, and/or cortex. Consequently the neuromuscular characteristics and perceptual characteristics of their speech production will be determined by the portions of the nervous system damaged. Constellations of perceptual features typically associated with multiple sclerosis (Darley, Brown, and Goldstein, 1972) and Wilson's disease (Berry, Darley, Aronson, and Goldstein, 1974) have been described.

Coexistence of Disorders. Aphasia, dysarthria, apraxia, and behavioral disturbances associated with right brain damage and chronic and acute organic brain syndromes are not mutually exclusive. In fact, a patient who exhibits several of these disorders at the same time is perhaps more common than a patient with only a singular communicative disorder due to brain damage. Looking at one of the classification systems for aphasia will easily provide an example of this. Two of the categories developed by

Schuell et al. (1964) include patients with generalized intellectual deterioration and dysarthria associated with aphasia.

Correlates of Brain Damage. Brain damage produces sensory, motor, psychosocial, and emotional deficits in addition to communicative impairments. Motor impairment affects mobility and self-help skills of everyday living. The patient may have difficulty walking, dressing, and eating. The sensory impairments may have been premorbid degenerative changes in vision and audition but now gain added importance because they reduce further the residual communicative skills of the patient.

The emotional and psychosocial reactions of the patient must not necessarily be considered pathologic or unexpected. Patients experience fear because they have had a close encounter with death; anger because they thought this only happened to others, not them; frustration because they find themselves unable to perform tasks previously handled with ease; and guilt because they feel they have become a burden rather than an asset to those around them. Patients may become increasingly dependent on their family and friends in order to elicit a demonstration of continued emotional attachment. Patients may also exhibit catastrophic reactions because they can no longer deal with stressful situations and respond by emotional outbursts of anger and crying.

The family is also dramatically affected. The major economic support of the family may be lost. Parenting may now be left to a single person rather than to a couple. The spouse who may have enjoyed a dependency role in the family is now required to cope not only with the economic and emotional demands of children but also with a husband or wife who requires a great deal of emotional support. The disruption in family life frequently occurs at a time when it has the greatest impact on financial and emotional resources.

Both patients and families will need to make adjustments if problems resulting from nervous system pathology are to be improved. Patients must recognize that the problems are long-term, that complete recovery is seldom, if ever, possible, and that rehabilitation is a difficult and arduous task. Families must recognize the seriousness of patients' sensory, motor, communicative, and emotional problems and provide continued support through the rehabilitation process.

SUMMARY

This chapter has reviewed the neurological bases of speech and language, the etiologies of nervous system impairment, and characteristics of neurogenic communicative disorders. It has also reviewed, albeit very briefly, some frequent concomitants of brain damage that have an impact on the rehabilitation process. Given this information, the next step is to describe instruments that serve as measures of the disorders and that aid in establishing what problems are to be treated.

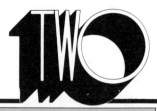

○ INTRODUCTION

○ TEST BATTERIES FOR APHASIA AND RELATED DISORDERS

○ OTHER TESTS FOR NEUROGENIC DISORDERS

○ PROCEDURES FOR ASSESSING NEUROMOTOR DISORDERS

○ EXAMINER AND PATIENT VARIABILITY

○ CONTEXT

○ DIFFERENTIAL DIAGNOSIS

aphasia

apraxia

dysarthria

confusion and dementia

○ CLINICAL EXAMPLES

○ SUMMARY

The evaluation

○ INTRODUCTION

Identification includes appraisal and diagnosis. *Appraisal* implies calibrated observation and measurement. *Measurement* requires obtaining direct quantitative data, and *test batteries* and *assessment protocols* are primary vehicles for obtaining behavioral observations. *Diagnosis* consists of placing the behavioral observations into context with the rest of the information available from the patient so that the disorder can be differentiated from other disorders having similar characteristics. *Differential diagnosis* is the assignment of a label to a group of behaviors that have been observed and quantified. The identification process then has three important components: test batteries and assessment protocols that serve as instruments for quantifying communicative behaviors; the context and perspective of the patient provided by medical, familial, social, and vocational histories; and the differential diagnosis of the disorder based upon the information available from assessment and contextual sources. Each of these processes will be considered with the understanding that a rationale for the process is important to gaining an understanding of the value of the information obtained.

○ TEST BATTERIES FOR APHASIA AND RELATED DISORDERS

Test batteries for neurogenic disorders have evolved from divergent rationales and reflect the fact that there are no universally accepted definitions or descriptions for communicative disorders arising from brain damage. Moreover, no test at present is so potent an aid to description or quantification of communicative behaviors that it supersedes all others in value or use. Benton (1967) addressed some of the problems in test construction for aphasia and compared their stage of development to intelligence tests available before the pioneering work of Binet. By that he meant that batteries had been developed for assessing neurogenic disorders, but they were insufficiently standardized and had not gained broad usage. Additionally he noted that the batteries were based upon preconceived theoretical assumptions regarding the characteristics of neurogenic communication disorders, assumptions that were agreed upon by only a limited number of clinicians.

Since Benton's observations on aphasia testing, several tests have been developed which have at least partially answered his standardization critique. On the other hand, preconceived notions remain regarding the characteristics and classifications of the communicative disorders resulting from brain damage. Test batteries for neurogenic disorders will be reviewed to point out their constructional adequacies and to describe the rationale from which the testmakers began.

Definitions of disorders identified by the tests will also be presented to serve as examples of classification systems available. However no direct attempt will be made to argue the relative merits of disorder categories proposed or to examine the equivalence of deficits encompassed under particular labels. The emphasis clearly will be on the instruments of appraisal.

Aphasia assessment batteries have a number of common features. Each (1) attempts to describe deficits in reading, writing, speaking, and understanding; (2) has items within a subtest and/or subtests within the battery arranged in a hierarchy based on difficulty; (3) provides information on interpretation of results; and (4) alludes to the necessity of providing information of a qualitative type regarding the responses obtained. At the same time they differ significantly in rationale, interpretation, scoring, and comprehensiveness.

Examining for Aphasia (Eisenson, 1954) was developed on the premise that aphasic disturbances are impairments in the patient's ability to handle situations involving internal symbol processes (thinking) and external symbol processes (speaking, reading, writing). The battery, containing 16 subtests designed to assess subsymbolic and symbolic abilities, is divided into two parts: items used to evaluate simple recognition and evaluation (predominantly receptive) and items used to evaluate expressive and productive skills (predominantly expressive). Deficits in recognition are defined as *agnosias;* disorders of evaluation and expression as *aphasias;* and deficits in production as *apraxias.*

The items in each subtest are arranged in order of increasing difficulty, and the test attempts to obtain a maximal performance from the patient under ideal conditions. Specific procedures are provided for administering each item, but only general directions are provided on several subtests because the examiner may have to determine the optimal means of presentation. Scoring is primarily dichotomous, but behaviors, response times, and modifications of administrative procedures are recorded.

The examiner may accept a variety of possible responses as long as the response signifies understanding of the item. The test has not been standardized, and no scale of percentage scores or other weighting is provided. In fact, Eisenson observed that it was not ". . . likely that a standardized test for aphasics can be produced which would permit a clinician to measure percentage of loss as a whole or even to estimate accurately percentage of loss within a given area of language function. Aphasic patients are characteristically too inconsistent in their responses to permit formal scoring standards to be developed and meaningfully applied" (p. 31). The degree of deficit relative to each symbol function area is estimated from the patient's performance and categorized as complete, severe, moderate, little, or none. Subtest performances are therefore used to estimate the presence and severity of aphasic, apractic, and agnosic disturbances. The test can be shortened by administering only every other item, and presentation of only the first item of each subtest constitutes a screening examination.

Several points need to be made about the rationale and usefulness of this test battery. First, the battery is based on a theoretical premise that receptive and expressive symbolic disorders can be differentiated, a point of view derived from the work of Weisenburg and McBride (1935) whose classification is a modified form of a dichotomous concept of aphasia and one that has not held up well under careful scrutiny. Second, the test purports to identify and quantify agnosias (recognition disturbances), deficits that are difficult to recognize because they share many behavioral characteristics with aphasia. Finally, even though the test is an avowedly clinical instrument, it does not negate the need for standardization to determine the reliability and validity of the measure. When viewed in historical perspective, *Examining for Aphasia* is allied with the theoretical constructs of Weisenburg and McBride (1935) and with early tests of aphasia that were not standardized.

The Language Modalities Test of Aphasia (Wepman and Jones, 1961) purportedly provides a psycholinguistic analysis of the aphasic patients' language and is based on the performance of more than 200 adult aphasic patients. Factor analysis of the data (Jones and Wepman, 1961) led the authors to posit two roles for language in the central nervous system: transmissive functions producing nonsymoblic language processes and integrative functions producing symbolic comprehension and formulation processes. They suggested that dysfunction of the modality-bound transmissive functions resulted in agnosias and apraxias and that integration dysfunctions produced aphasias.

The test consists of two forms comparable in difficulty which are presented on filmstrips 120 frames in length. The two forms of the test allow test-retest evaluations as a means of measuring the stability of the performance of the patient. The initial items on each form of the test are identical and constitute a screening section. Five different types of responses are elicited from the patient: oral, graphic, and three types of matching. Dichotomous scoring is used for the screening section and the standardized visual- and auditory-matching items. For the oral and graphic responses and storytelling sections, the responses are scored on a six-point scale and identified as normal, syntactic, semantic, pragmatic, jargon, or global. The results of testing are summarized, and the patient is classified according to one of the available categories: pragmatic, semantic, syntactic, jargon or global aphasia, and apraxia and/or agnosia. The test battery has not been standardized.

The diagnostic categories of Wepman and Jones are shown in Table 2-1. Examination of the table reveals basic similarities between Wepman and

TABLE 2–1

Classification, Definition and Description of Aphasia from the
Language Modalities Test for Aphasia

TYPE	DEFINITION	CHARACTERISTICS
Pragmatic	A disorder of comprehension of symbols in which the patient fails to associate incoming signals with appropriate concepts.	Patients convey little meaning in their speech. They are constricted in their vocabularies, using fewer low frequency words than would be expected in light of their premorbid education and vocation. They show an excessive use of neologisms, meaningless verbal efforts apparently substituted for specific substantive words. They have inadequate feedback along all modalities, rarely recognizing their errors or their inability to communicate satisfactorily. Not infrequently they substitute or insert inappropriate substantive words. However they are able to maintain a flow of language, they retain the melody and pitch changes of normal speech, and they do not deviate appreciably from the normal in terms of relative frequency of usage of the various parts of speech.
Semantic	Disorder of symbol formulation in which the patient has difficulty attaching a meaningful verbal sign to a previously acquired concept; impairment of the ability to recall and use previously acquired verbal forms applicable to such a concept.	Patients have great difficulty remembering and using once familiar proper names or substantive words (i.e., nouns, verbs, adjectives) except, possibly, the most frequent and general; when trying to recall words of this type, they frequently employ pauses, hesitation forms, repetition, or phrases indicating their inability to recall; in place of a word which they cannot recall, they sometimes employ circumlocutions or vocal and body gestures. However they retain the use of the highly frequent function words (articles, demonstratives, pronouns, prepositions) and, often, highly frequent substantive words. To a large extent they retain the flow, the melody and pitch changes, and the grammatical structure of normal speech except when interrupted or deflected by their inability to recall and use a desired word.
Syntactic	A disorder of symbol formulation in which the patient is unable to use his or her previously acquired grammatical structure.	Patients tend to misuse and, more often, omit altogether the function words (i.e., articles, demonstratives, pronouns, prepositions, auxiliary verbs) and therefore cannot form sentences or smaller syntactic constructions, such as prepositional phrases, noun phrases, or verb phrases, but speak telegraphically using single substantive words. They retain little of the melody of speech although rising and falling pitch are used accompanying single words. However they retain many substantive words (nouns, verbs, adjectives) and often retain automatic phrases and a very few minimal sentence types.
Jargon	A disorder of symbol formulation and expression in	Patients almost exclusively use sequences of phonemes which are unlike any specific words

26

TABLE 2-1 (Continued)

TYPE	DEFINITION	CHARACTERISTICS
	which previously acquired sequences of phonemes making up intelligible units of speech are no longer available, and unintelligible ones (i.e., jargon) are used in their stead.	of their previously acquired language but which generally follow the overall phonemic patterns of that language (i.e., its consonants, vowels, and their permitted combinations), as well as its accentual and pitch patterns, suggesting that their attempts at language may be meaningful to them. As recall for recognizable words improves, the patients appear most like one or the other of the types previously described. However the most frequent words of the language and the syntax are more often recovered than are substantive words. Jargon expressions often are retained as neologisms after comparatively complete recovery.
Global	A disorder of language in which the patient either is unable to respond verbally to stimuli or responds with an automatized word, phrase, or phoneme sequence.	Patients evidence little or no understanding along any modality and little or no ability to communicate. Comprehension, where it exists at all, is generally limited to specific immediate concerns of the patient. Patients may often rely on primitive gesture and facial expressions to indicate their needs. In some, there is evident retention of a meaningful automatic phrase or word. Sometimes the use is appropriate, and sometimes it is so automatic that it is indiscriminant.
Agnosia	Failure of incoming signals to arouse a meaningful state due to transmission defects attending a specific stimulus modality evidenced by the inability to imitate, copy, or recognize stimuli or to match them with identical stimuli.	Disruptions of the reception of language stimuli where the transmission function of the central nervous system is affected rather than the integrative function which produces the symbolic formulation of the language. Disorder specific to stimulus modalities—a disruption of a particular transmission pathway has no necessary relationship to disruption of input along any other modality. The effect on total language of an agnosia is largely on the reception of stimuli along the modality concerned. The capacity to formulate symbols is often found to be little affected. Specific islands of ability are often retained. Description requires specification of modality, type of loss, and degree of loss within each type.
Apraxia	A disruption in the ability to transmit or express a motor response along a specific modality; difficulty in the articulation of speech, in the formation of letters in writing, or in the movements of gesture or pantomime. Includes all of the specific motor defects from the most central disorders where the actual recall of motor positioning and sequencing of speech articulators are af-	Verbal apraxia is the loss of ability to produce the motor acts of articulation at will. The disorder is independent of the symbolic process. The patient understands what is said, formulates symbols, has available the syntax of the language, but cannot recall or control the motor act of articulation. In writing, the same independence of disability is seen. However verbal and agraphic apraxias are independent of one another. The dysarthrias are varieties of verbal apraxia. The nature of the dysarthric problem depends upon the location of the neural disability. Central dysarthria not only affects articulation in speed of movement and

TABLE 2-1 (Continued)

TYPE	DEFINITION	CHARACTERISTICS
	fected to the various levels and degrees of dysarthria and agraphia.	consequent elision and omission of sounds produced or attempted but also produces reversals of sounds and syllables within words and between words as well as substitution of phonetic patterns. The more distal disturbances in articulation, the peripheral dysarthrias, show only the problem of speech articulation without the reversals and substitutions. They typically show elongated vowels and slow articulation.

Adapted from J. Weppman and L. Jones, *The Language Modalities Test for Aphasia*, Chicago: Education-Industry Service, 1961. Reprinted by permission.

Jones and Eisenson: their recognition and acceptance of the idea that agnosias and apraxias are modality bound coexistent disorders to aphasia and their consistency in conceiving of language as a hierarchically arranged symbolic function. Wepman and Jones, however, view aphasia as a regressive linguistic disorder with comparable and recognizable stages in childhood language acquisition, an ontogenetic regression hypothesis which cannot withstand the weight of more recent linguistic studies of aphasia (see Caramazza and Zurif, 1978). From the point of view of rationale, the adequacy of the test is reduced in value because it is yoked to the ontogenetic retrogression hypothesis. From the standpoint of clinical utility, its value is reduced by the lack of standardization.

The *Minnesota Test for the Differential Diagnosis of Aphasia* (Schuell, 1965) is similar to *Examining for Aphasia* and the *Language Modalities Test of Aphasia* in that aphasia is viewed as a unitary disorder which may be complicated by other communicative deficits. It is clearly different in its assignment of the patient to one of five major and two minor categories or syndromes based upon prognostically valuable patterns of impairment. The test contains 47 subtests divided into five areas: auditory disturbances, visual and reading disturbances, speech and language disturbances, visuomotor and writing disturbances, and disturbances of numerical relations and arithmetic processes. The patient's responses to test items are primarily dichotomously scored. The patient is assigned to one of five major or two minor categories based on subtest performance. The major groups include simple aphasia, aphasia with visual involvement, aphasia with sensorimotor involvement, aphasia with scattered findings compatible with generalized brain damage, and irreversible aphasic syndrome. The two minor syndromes are aphasia with partial auditory imperception and aphasia with persisting dysarthria (Table 2-2).

In addition to factor analysis of the scores from 157 aphasic subjects, means, standard deviations, median scores, and percentage of subjects making errors are provided for each subtest. However no standard scores or numerical indices of severity are provided because Schuell (1965) rejected them as "... meaningless when dealing with aphasic populations which are heterogeneous in age, intelligence, cultural milieu, medical history, locus and extent of brain damage, and severity and duration of aphasia" (p. 7). She also stated that "... the most effective way of interpreting test data is in terms of clinical signs and total test pattern" (p. 8).

A short version of the test, intended for screening, has been developed (Schuell, 1957) and reevaluated (Schuell, 1966). Diagnostic and severity rating scales are also included in the complete test battery.

The *Minnesota Test for the Differential Diagnosis of Aphasia* has no clearcut theoretical basis other than the notion that aphasia is a singular disorder. Its premise is clearly based on the need for descriptive clinical testing because description helps determine both prognosis and treatment in aphasia.

The necessity for pragmatic description of patient deficits and residual functions also is reflected in the *Functional Communication Profile* (Sarno, 1969). Sarno observed that most clinical tests for aphasia do not consider that many aphasic patients use gestures to communicate, respond accurately but inconsistently, require a longer period of time to respond even when vocabulary and syntax are intact, and have more difficulty with highly specific tasks. She also indicated that many of the more standard aphasia batteries are relatively insensitive to minimal impairments and may contain many items to which the severely involved patient cannot respond. The Functional Communication Profile is a rating scale that specifies everyday performance and is not limited to stimulus response behavioral paradigms in a clinical test situation. It is an adjunct to stimulus response test batteries, not a substitute. The test is a descriptive device and does not address issues such as symptomatology, diagnostic categories, reasons for patients not using a particular behavior, or therapy rationales.

The scale consists of 45 integrated communicative behaviors divided into five areas based upon a factor analysis: movement, speaking, understanding, reading, and miscellaneous (including writing and calculation). Ratings of each behavior are made on a continuum along a nine-point scale from zero to normal and considers the speed, accuracy, consistency, voluntary control without benefit of external cues, and compensatory function of the behavior. Ideally the ratings would be based on direct observation of the patient in communicative situations throughout the day. More typically they are made following informal interaction with the patient in an interview, supplemented, when necessary, by reports from family members and other professionals working with the patient. The ratings are based on *what* the patient does, not on *how well* the activities are performed. The ratings from the five sections and the entire profile are converted to percentages which reflect the percent of premorbid or "normal" functioning. A patient rated as functioning at the 80th percentile, for example, would be estimated to be function-

TABLE 2-2

Characteristics and Prognosis of Aphasic Syndromes Identified by the Minnesota Test for the Differential Diagnosis of Aphasia

GROUP	DESIGNATION	CHARACTERISTICS	PROGNOSIS
I	Simple Aphasia	Reduction of language in all modalities in the absence of any specific visual, motor, or sensorimotor impairment. Usually word-finding problems are present, with the most common error being substitution of a word associated in meaning with the intended word. Those with a moderate or moderately severe impairment show frequent inconsistent mispronunciations. In some patients, speech is unintelligible or jargonic. Impairment is related to disturbances in the auditory feedback mechanisms and the impaired recall of learned auditory patterns. Auditory comprehension is usually good for short units, but errors increase as materials increase in length. Writing is similar to oral expression.	Excellent
II	Aphasia with Cerebral Involvement of Visual Processes	Mild to severe language impairment in all modalities characterized by a reduction of vocabulary and verbal retention. Pattern of impairment similar to Group I with the addition of impaired visual processing in the recognition and recall of learned visual patterns which affect both reading and writing. Impaired visual processes include the confusion of visual symbols with similar configurations due to the inability to make fine visual discriminations.	Excellent for language not dependent on visual processes. Recovery is slowest in reading and writing.
III	Aphasia with Sensorimotor Involvement	Reduction of language in all modalities with some inconsistency due to difficulty producing the learned movement patterns required for speech in the absence of observable paralysis or paresis of the speech musculature. Articulation is defective and the automaticity of speech is lost. Articulation errors are usually consistent in pattern. The sounds that require complicated movement patterns usually are more defective than those with simple ones; groups of consonants and consonant blends are more defective than single ones, and polysyllabic words are more defective than monosyllabic ones.	Limited, but a functional recovery of language is possible.

IV	Asphasia with Visual and Motor Involvement	Reduction of vocabulary and verbal retention span is reflected in all language modalities. Mild to severe language impairment is present, but residual functional language in one modality or another always remains. Errors in reading and writing are present. Writing quality is generally poor. Some blurring or intermittent clouding or vision and spatial disorientation may be present. Almost always some motor involvement of the speech musculature such as paresis or paralysis.	Not as much improvement possible as can be attained by Groups I, II, and III. However therapy is still indicated.
V	Irreversible Aphasia Syndrome	Almost a complete loss of functional language skills in all modalities. More errors on all functions than members of any other group. Errors are made in pointing to common objects and in following simple directions. Patients may, however, be able to match a few words to pictures. Neither reading nor writing is functional.	Poor prognosis since gains made do not become functional. Only limited and realistic short-term therapy is indicated.
Minor Aphasic Syndrome A	Aphasia with Partial Auditory Imperception and Some Residual Language Retained or Recovered Early	A relatively severe deficit is present in all language modalities. Auditory imperception is always partial. Although verbal output is high, little information is conveyed.	Uncertain, but a gradual and consistent recovery of language is usually achieved.
Minor Asphasic Syndrome B	Mild Aphasia with Persisting Dysarthria	Speech is hesitant and slurred with many errors of articulation. Articulatory errors increase in relationship to message length and speech rate. Sibilants are more involved than other consonants.	Good recovery from aphasia with the probability that good articulation can be achieved.

Adapted from L. Sies, ed., *Aphasia Theory and Therapy: Selected Lectures and Papers of Hildred Schuell*. Baltimore: University Park Press (1974). Reprinted by permission.

ing at 80 percent of premorbid level. Premorbid capacity consequently is a reference against which the performance of the patient is measured. The profile of the patient can also be used to visually differentiate between types of communicative impairment. For example, if a patient demonstrates severely impaired speaking skills compared to rated performance on other sections of the scale, he or she might be described as demonstrating verbal apraxia.

In contrast to tests discussed earlier, the Functional Communication Profile stands out as an evaluation instrument which attempts to determine communicative abilities in "typical" everyday situations rather than obtaining maximal performance under ideal conditions. It carries with it no preconceived assumptions regarding classifications of aphasia or localization of lesions.

The *Neurosensory Center Comprehensive Examination of Aphasia* (Spreen and Benton, 1969) is another eclectically derived instrument without stated concern with types of aphasia. The test consists of 20 tests of language performance and 4 tests of visual and tactile function. The 20 language tests assess language comprehension and production, retention of verbal information, and reading and writing. The four visual and tactile function tests are designed to detect deficits in these skills and are administered whenever a patient's performance on tests such as visual or tactile naming is subnormal. Dichotomous scoring is used, although incorrect and mispronounced correct responses are also recorded and any unusual features of performance noted.

This battery is unique because it provides for construction of a profile of directly comparable percentile scores corrected for age and educational level. Two profile sheets have been developed for this purpose. The first profile is based on the performance of normal adults on the battery. The raw scores are computed for each of the 20 language tests, corrected for age and educational level (where appropriate), and transformed into the corresponding percentile rank of a normal population. Benton and Spreen suggest that patients without language deficits will perform at the 40th percentile or above. Performance at the 30th to 40th percentile suggests minimal difficulty; at the 20th to 30th percentile, mild impairment, and below the 20th percentile, more severe dysfunction. The second profile compares the patient's performance with a reference group of aphasic patients. Thus the patient's strengths and weaknesses can be determined relative to the "average" performance of other aphasic patients. The profile presents a configuration of residual abilities and is interpreted without using a classification for different types of aphasia, although Benton (1967) has presented patterns for patients referred with various diagnoses such as "jargon aphasia," "anomia," "Gerstmann's syndrome," and "expressive aphasia."

⨈ The *Porch Index of Communicative Ability* (Porch, 1967, 1971), designed to assess verbal, gestural, and graphic abilities, is based on the premise that two major requirements of an aphasia examination are high reliability and a scoring system which specifies the nature of the patient's response in terms of multiple dimensions. The test contains 18 subtests (four verbal, eight gestural, and six graphic), each having ten items. The responses to the 180 items of the test are scored according to a 16-point binary choice system which considers the accuracy, responsiveness, completeness, promptness, and efficiency of the response. Mean scores for each subtest, each modality, and the entire battery are computed from the 180 responses. The mean subtest scores can be examined on a modality response summary which contains a plotting of scores by modality and a ranked response summary on which the means are plotted in order of decreasing subtest difficulty.

The Porch index was standardized on 280 patients with left hemisphere damage and 100 bilaterally brain-damaged patients. Percentiles are provided for each subtest and modality, for the entire battery, and for the mean of the nine high and nine low subtests. The nine high, nine low, and overall test means are used to plot a recovery curve for the patient. The recovery curve is used to make predictions regarding the patient's eventual communicative functioning based on the performance at one month post onset. At six months the mean of the patient's nine high subtests is considered the best estimate of his or her eventual maximal level of recovery. Five types of profiles are identified based on test results: (1) aphasia without complications, (2) aphasia complicated by verbal formulation or verbal expression problems, (3) aphasia patterns with accompanying illiteracy, (4) bilateral brain damage, and (5) aberrant patterns suggesting that the communicative disorder is not aphasia.

A large data base has been acquired for the index since the original standardization by Porch. Duffy, Keith, Shane, and Podraza (1976) provided subtest, modality, and overall test scores for 130 normal, nonbrain-injured adults, and Watson and Records (1978) investigated the effectiveness of the test in assessing specific behaviors in senile dementia. The test has been criticized for its lack of ordinality (McNeil, Prescott, and Chang, 1975) and specification of the response, neglect of factors related to communication, distortions in modality scoring, inadequacies of the response categories, statistical treatment of scores, and conceptual limits (Martin, 1977). It should be recognized, however, that almost any of the standardized test batteries could be criticized on some of the same parameters.

The Porch index is unique because of its multidimensional scoring system, the rigidity with which items are administered, the detailed statistical analysis of subject performances for standardization, and the requirement of 40 hours of training to develop competency in administration. It is not purported to be of significant value in localizing the site of lesion, although recovery curves may be used to estimate the type of lesion. The instrument then is basically a descriptive device without major assumptions regarding classifications of aphasia.

✶ *The Boston Diagnostic Aphasia Examination* (Goodglass and Kaplan, 1972) is based on the assumption that the aphasic deficit is determined by "a. the anatomical organization of language in the brain, b. the location of the causative lesion, and c. the functional interactions (e.g., inhibitory, regulatory, selective) of various parts of the language system" (p. 2). According to Goodglass and Kaplan, the test battery is geared toward determining the type of aphasic syndrome in order to infer the site of lesion, to measure communicative and related skills for initial description, and to detect change in performance over time. The test also provides a comprehensive assessment of abilities and deficits that can serve as a therapy guide.

The battery contains 23 subtests used to assess auditory comprehension, oral expression, reading and writing, ratings of six speech characteristics (melodic line, phrase length, articulatory agility, grammatical form, paraphasia, and word finding) on a seven-point, equal-interval scale and a rating of severity on a six-point scale based on a sample of conversational and expository speech, plus 13 language and 14 nonlanguage subtests. Scoring on the subtests is primarily dichotomous with some longhand notation.

The battery was standardized on 207 aphasic patients. Based on the range, mean, and standard deviation of their performances, Z scores were computed so that the patient's performance on each subtest can be compared with the standardization population in standard deviation units. Based on the rating scale profile of speech characteristics and Z scores, the patient may be assigned to one of several diagnostic categories, including Broca's aphasia, Wernicke's aphasia, anomic aphasia, conduction aphasia, transcortical sensory and motor aphasias, and alexia with agraphia (Table 2–3). The supplementary tests, most of which lack statistical norms, explore psycholinguistic factors in auditory comprehension and verbal expression, repetition disorders, tests of disconnection syndromes, a "parietal lobe" battery, and tests for nonverbal apraxia.

The Boston test is unique in that it uses behavioral characteristics to localize the site of lesion. This classical orientation to aphasia is at variance with the assumptions of earlier testmakers such as Schuell and Wepman and Jones. However the differences between these tests are not in the areas of communication assessed or in the behaviors observed but in the inferences that are drawn from the test results—a bias not easily surmounted since the inference is always judgmental.

The *Western Aphasia Battery* (Kertesz & Poole, 1974) bears a close resemblance to the *Boston Diagnostic Aphasia Examination.* Kertesz (1978) noted that some of the Western subtests incorporate material from the Boston test; therefore similarities in the test structure and content are to be expected. However the Western battery varies from the Boston in that results are expressed as quotients rather than Z scores. Spontaneous speech, comprehension, repetition, and naming subtest scores are used to calculate an aphasia quotient (AQ) and to describe the type and severity of aphasia. Reading, writing, praxis (gestures), drawing, block design, calculation and the Raven Progressive Matrices test performances are used to compute a performance quotient (PQ), which if combined with the AQ yields a cortical quotient (CQ). Performance on the naming, fluency, comprehension, and repetition measures allow assignment of the patient to one of eight aphasia types: global, Broca's, isolation, transcortical motor, Wernicke's, anomic, transcortical sensory, or conduction. Criteria for aphasia-type assignment was based on the performance of 150 aphasic patients in an initial standardization sample. The AQ also can be used to separate aphasic from neurologically normal patients but not from neurologically impaired nonaphasic patients, based on a later standardization. Shewan and Kertesz (1980) documented the reliability and validity of the Western Battery.

The Aphasia Language Performance Scales (Keenan & Brassell, 1975) were developed because the authors believed that existing aphasia tests had several unsatisfactory conditions: They were time consuming, were limited by space and environmental restrictions, tended to break down rapport, and gave little help in planning for therapy. The test is composed of four scales (listening, talking, reading, writing), each containing ten items. The items on each scale are graded in difficulty and range in linguistic complexity from virtual absence of function to near-normal function. The four scales are purported to be independent of one another—that is, performance on items of one scale are not affected by deficits tested by items from another scale.

Each item is scored one point if the response is correct or self-corrected, one-half point if the response is corrected following prompting, and zero points for an incorrect response. The score on each scale is computed and plotted on a summary form which can be used to illustrate the patient's pattern of impairment, severity of the deficit in each modality, and rate of improvement. The test must be viewed as a pragmatic clinical screening tool which attempts to describe the performance of the aphasic adult but which is not concerned with the classifications of aphasia or theoretical frameworks typically employed to differentiate types of aphasia.

Communicative Abilities in Daily Life (Holland, 1979; 1980) is a 68-item test instrument which emphasizes a functional approach to assessing the patient's communicative impairment. Holland noted that the primary focus is on whether the message was completed, not on whether it was communicated by verbal or nonverbal means. Consequently the test is not modality specific. The Communicative Abilities Scale has a three-point scoring system. If the patient's response was successful whether by verbal, gestural, or graphic means, it is considered correct and scored two. If it was not totally correct but signified a communicative relationship to the task item, it is scored as one. If it was failed, it is scored as zero. Items on the test are

TABLE 2–3

Aphasia Classification from Boston Diagnostic Aphasia Examination

TYPE	SITE OF LESION	CHARACTERISTICS
Wernicke's Aphasia	Posterior portion of the first temporal gyrus.	Impaired auditory comprehension and fluently articulated but paraphasic speech. Patient may repeat words uncomprehendingly or with literal or verbal paraphasia. In severe forms paraphasia may be so pervasive that oral expression is meaningless jargon. Word-finding problems are a constant feature of the disorder. Reading and writing are usually severely impaired. Grammer is often correct but with few departures from simple declarative word order. Repetition is fluent but paraphasic with neologisms. Rate of speech production may be increased.
Broca's Aphasia	Third frontal convolution.	Awkward articulation, restricted vocabulary, restriction of grammar to the simplest, most overlearned forms and relative preservation of auditory comprehension. Written language follows the pattern of speech in that writing is usually at least as severely impaired as speech, while reading is only mildly affected. Nonspeech oral movements are often, *but not always*, affected.
Anomic Aphasia	Temporal-parietal region—may extend to angular gyrus.	Major feature is the prominence of word-finding difficulty in the context of fluent, grammatically well-formed speech. Differs from Wernicke's aphasia in the absence of literal and verbal paraphasia and in the relative intactness of auditory comprehension. Patient may use circumlocutions in free speech. Conversation strikingly free of content words. Significantly poorer comprehension of isolated nouns and verbs with respect to their overall comprehension level than demonstrated by other types of patients. Reading and writing may vary in severity over a wide range from patient to patient. Least reliably localized of the aphasias—no sharp demarcation from Wernicke's aphasia; rather, appears there is a continuum from Wernicke's to anomic.
Conduction Aphasia	Supramarginal gyrus deep to arcuate fasciculus.	Repetition is disproportionately severely impaired in relation to the level of fluency in spontaneous speech and to the near-normal level of auditory comprehension. Spontaneous speech may be circumlocutory and inadequately structured with defective syntax and difficulty finding words appropriate to a context. Defects of structure and gross misspelling characterize writing. Reading near normal limits. Outstanding speech difficulty is in the proper choice and sequencing of phonemes so that literal paraphasia constantly interferes with production—especially during repetition.

TABLE 2-3 (Continued)

TYPE	SITE OF LESION	CHARACTERISTICS
	Band of infarcted tissue which cuts off an intact Wernicke-Broca area from rest of the brain.	Remarkable preservation of repetition in the context of the features of a severe Wernicke's aphasia. Patient does not initiate speech. When addressed, speech is well articulated with irrelevant paraphasia and neologisms. Totally unable to name when confronted, but usually offers grossly irrelevant responses when so stimulated. May be echolalia, but repetition not limited to echoing since patient may be able to repeat sentences of considerable length and complexity. Unusual preservation of memorized material. Reading and writing severely involved.
Transcortical Motor Aphasia	Tissue of frontal lobe marginal to third frontal gyrus.	Marked by absence of spontaneous speech and writing, although can reply briefly to questions. Confrontation naming relatively intact. Difficulty in initiating and organizing response, but once initiated, it is well articulated. Auditory comprehension, oral reading, repetition, and writing to dictation are relatively preserved.

Adapted from H. Goodglass, & E. Kaplan, *The assessment of aphasia and other disorders*. Philadelphia: Lea and Febiger, 1972. Used by permission.

". . . everyday tasks ranging from responding to and giving social greetings to differentiating nonverbal signs on restroom doors to comprehending metaphors to recognizing statements which are contextually absurd and unpredictable" (1979, p. 15). The items are encompassed within ". . . simulated, real-world activities, including going to the doctor's office, riding in a car, shopping, using the telephone and being interviewed by a stranger" (1979, p. 15). The total score is the cumulative sum of the item scores.

The test is of particular interest because of its attempt to identify and quantify the communicative impairment of the patient in activities more analogous to those in which the patient would normally participate. Standardization of the test also revealed that

> Overall communicative strengths and deficits were . . . not discriminated by pattern of performance in different modalities. Rather, all modalities appeared to reflect the extent to which the entire communicative system was compromised by aphasia. (1980, p. 29)

Interestingly this finding is similar to Schuell et al.'s who noted that aphasia is a unitary disorder which may be complicated by other deficits but is primarily defined by the severity of the linguistic deficit.

In this section many, but by no means all, of the aphasia batteries designed to evaluate communicative skills have been reviewed. Other tests include the *Halstead Aphasia Test, Form M* (Halstead, Wepman, Reitan, &

Heimburger, undated), The *Orzeck Aphasia Evaluation* (Orzeck, 1964), and the *Sklar Aphasia Scale* (Sklar, 1966). Perhaps the overriding commonality of all the tests described is the emphasis on *description* and *quantification* of communicative disorders in the areas of auditory comprehension, verbal expression, reading, and writing. Beyond this common feature, they go their separate ways as results are used to make prognoses, plan therapy, or predict the site of lesion. A summary of the test batteries for aphasia and related disorders reviewed are presented in Table 2–4.

A clinical example may help to point out interpretative similarities and differences in aphasia test battery results. Patient S., 21 years old, suffered a large-caliber, perforating missile wound to the head. The point of entry was mid-low forehead, and exit was the left temporal parietal region. A left frontotemporal craniotomy was performed with debridement of the wound. It was noted during this procedure that the missile had destroyed the pre-frontal lobe, Broca's area, anterior portions of the first and second temporal gyri, and branches of the middle cerebral artery. Computerized axial tomography performed 18 months post-onset revealed a large low-density area consistent with encephalomalacia in the distribution of the left anterior cerebral artery and anterior aspect of the left middle cerebral artery. The lesion, then, included a large area of the frontal lobe and anterior temporal lobe.

For purposes of comparison, the patient was administered four test batteries more than 18 months post brain damage. The Porch Index of Communicative Ability (PICA) and Boston Diagnostic Aphasia Examination (BDAE) were administered to compare standardized measures of speech and language functioning; the Functional Communication Profile (FCP) and Communicative Abilities of Daily Living (CADL) were used to estimate performance in situations encompassed in everyday communicative interactions. Results of the tests will be examined rather broadly. Individual item analyses for the purpose of therapy planning will not be undertaken.

Results of the PICA are presented in Figure 2–1. Included are the score sheet, modality response summary, and ranked response summary. Shown on the score sheet are response levels for the ten items of the 18 subtests; overall, gestural, verbal and graphic modality means; and percentiles for these means based on a standardization sample of 280 left-brain-damaged aphasic subjects. Porch (1971) noted that the overall response level of 13.23 is indicative of patients who are reasonably adept at communication with little assistance. The 84 percent reflects the relatively better performance of Patient S. compared to the standardization population. Expected mean performance as a function of modality is 12.00, 10.00, and 8.00 for gestural, verbal, and graphic modalities, respectively (Porch, 1971). S.'s more intact ability in the graphic modality is revealed by a higher response level (mean = 13.08; 93 percent) for this modality when compared to gestural (mean = 13.66; 73 percent) and verbal (mean = 12.60; 59 percent) modali-

TABLE 2-4

Description, Scoring, Norms, and Interpretation of Aphasia Test Batteries

TEST	DESCRIPTION	SCORING	NORMS	INTERPRETATION
EXAMINING FOR APHASIA (Eisenson, 1954)	Subtests dichotomized into primarily receptive and primarily expressive portions. Within each section, subtests divided into those designed to test for subsymbolic or low symbolic function (agnosias, apraxias) and those designed to evaluate high symbolic function (aphasias).	Plus-minus with some longhanded notation.	None.	Rating of presence and severity of aphasia, apraxia, and agnosia as revealed by subtest performance.
THE LANGUAGE MODALITIES TEST FOR APHASIA (Wepman and Jones 1961)	Eleven screening items and two sets of 23 items presented on filmstrips 120 frames in length designed to assess auditory comprehension, verbal expression, reading and writing skills, plus calculation.	Plus-minus for screening and auditory and visual matching items. Oral, graphic, and story-telling sections rated on a six-point scale according to predominant characteristics of the response.	Factor analysis of the responses of 168 aphasic patients.	Results used to assign patient to categories based upon predominant characteristics of the disorder; pragmatic, semantic, syntactic, jargon or global aphasia, and/or apraxia and/or agnosia.
MINNESOTA TEST FOR DIFFERENTIAL DIAGNOSIS OF APHASIA (Schuell, 1965)	Fifty-seven subtests divided into five major sections: auditory disturbances, visual and reading disturbances, speech and language disturbances, visuomotor and writing disturbances, disturbances of numerical relations and arithmetic processes. Also includes clinical and severity rating scales and screening version.	Plus-minus with some longhand notation.	Means, standard deviations, median scores, percentages of 157 subjects making errors on each subtest.	Test score summarization and lists of signs and most discriminating tests used to assign patient to one of five major and two minor prognostic categories based on pattern of impairment.
FUNCTIONAL COMMUNICATION PROFILE (Sarno, 1969)	Forty-five integrated behaviors divided into movement, speaking, understanding, reading, and miscellaneous sections.	Behaviors rated on a nine-point rating scale.	None. However sample profiles presented.	Ratings converted to percentages for each section and test as a whole. Percentage purported to reflect residual communicative abilities compared to premorbid functioning.

TABLE 2–4 (Continued)

TEST	DESCRIPTION	SCORING	NORMS	INTERPRETATION
NEUROSENSORY CENTER COMPREHENSIVE EXAMINATION OF APHASIA (Spreen and Benton, 1969)	Twenty tests of language production and comprehension, retention of verbal information, reading, writing. Four tests of visual and tactile function.	Primarily plus-minus; some longhand notation.	Percentiles for each subtest from performance of neurologically normal and aphasic subjects. Number of subjects unspecified.	Some subtests corrected for age and education. Construction of subtest performance profiles to compare patient performance to that of normal and aphasic standardization populations.
PORCH INDEX OF COMMUNICATIVE ABILITY (Porch, 1967, 1971)	Four verbal, eight gestural, and six graphic subtests with ten items per subtest.	Responses scored according to 16-point binary choice system on the basis of accuracy, responsiveness, completeness, promptness, and efficiency.	Percentiles for the test as a whole, for each subtest, and for combinations of subtests by modality for 280 left hemisphere brain-damaged and 100 bilaterally brain-damaged subjects. Also percentiles for nine high, nine low, and overall scores. Examples of five basic performance patterns provided.	Overall and gestural, verbal and graphic modality means compared to standardization population and subtest scores plotted as a function of subtest difficulty. Also recovery curves determined by computation of nine high, nine low, and overall test means.
BOSTON DIAGNOSTIC APHASIA EXAMINATION (Goodglass and Kaplan, 1972)	Twenty-three subtests used to assess auditory comprehension, oral expression, reading, writing. Ratings of conversational and expository speech on six parameters and rating of severity. Also includes 13 language and 14 nonlanguage tests.	Primarily plus-minus with some longhand notation.	Z-score profiles based on the range, mean, and standard deviation of scores from 207 aphasic subjects. Intercorrelation analyses, and reliability coefficients among subtests also provided.	Overall severity on a six-point scale, speech characteristics ratings, and Z-score profiles used to assign patient to classical aphasic syndrome: Broca's aphasia, Wernicke's aphasia, anomic aphasia, conduction aphasia, transcortical sensory aphasia, transcortical motor aphasia, alexia without agraphia.

Test	Description	Scoring	Standardization	Comments
APHASIA LANGUAGE PERFORMANCE SCALES (Keenan and Brassell, 1975)	Four scales—listening, talking, reading, writing—each comprised of ten items.	One point per item if correct or self-corrected, one-half point if correct following prompt. No points if incorrect.	None.	Arbitrary assignments of scores from scales to degree of language impairment 0–1.0 profound 1.5–3.0 severe 3.5–5.0 moderate to severe 5.5–7.0 mild to moderate 7.5–9.0 mild 9.5–10.0 insignificant.
COMMUNICATIVE ABILITIES IN DAILY LIFE (Holland, 1980)	Sixty-eight items encompassed within simulated, real-world activities.	Two points if correct, one point if not totally correct but signifies a communicative relationship to the task item. No points if incorrect.	Means and standard deviations of scores from 130 neurologically normal and 130 aphasic subjects as a function of age, sex, institutionalization, and type of aphasia.	Total score is indication of communicative abilities during the course of every-day activities.
WESTERN APHASIA BATTERY (Kertesz and Poole, 1974).	Oral language subtests to appraise spontaneous speech, comprehension, repetition, and naming. Performance subtests to assess reading and writing, praxis and rhythm, and construction abilities (includes Raven Matrices).	Variable depending on subtest. Ranges from ten-point rating scales for functional content and fluency of spontaneous speech to dichotomous scoring of responses to read commands.	Means and standard deviations of fluency, comprehension, repetition, naming and information subtests, and aphasia quotients for 150 aphasics of various types and 59 nonbrain damaged, nondominant hemisphere brain-damaged, and brain-damaged nonaphasic patients (First Standardization). Means and standard deviations of subtests and aphasia quotients for 141 aphasics as a function of aphasia type and for 10 neurologically normal and 53 nondominant hemisphere brain-damaged patients (Second Standardization).	Oral language subtests and aphasia quotient used to determine type and severity of aphasia. Aphasia quotient also may be used to separate aphasic from neurologically normal patients.

Porch Index of Communicative Ability

BY BRUCE E. PORCH, PH.D.

SCORE SHEET

Name S.   Case No._____ Test No._____

Date 1/6/81   By jh   Time 12:35 to 1:15 Total Time 40 min.

Test Conditions Standard

Patient Conditions (R) used

TIME	12.35	12.38	12.41	12.43	12.45	12.46	12.48	12.51	12.52	12.54	12.55	12.57	1.00	1.03	1.05	1.07	1.10	1.12
ITEM	I	II	III	IV	V	VI	VII	VIII	IX	X	XI	XII	A	B	C	D	E	F
1. Tb	10(w)	15	11	10	15	15	9^5	15	15	15	15	15	5	14	14	15	15	14
2. Cg	11	7	7	15	15	15	15	15	15	15	15	15	7	15	15	15	10	15
3. Pn	(11)	12	12	10	15	15	15	15	10	15	15	15	5	15	15	15	15	15
4. Kf	5	9"	12	15	12	15	15	15	13	15	15	15	5	15	15	15	15	15
5. Fk	12	12	12	13	12	15	15	15	15	15	15	15	5	13	13	15	14	14
6. Qt	5	11	11	13	12	15	15	15	13	15	15	15	5	15	15	15	14	14
7. Pl	5	12	12	(13)	12	15	13	15	15	13	15	15	5	13	13	15	15	13
8. Mt	10(w)	12	12	(13)	12	15	15	15	11^r5	15	15	15	10	13	15	15	15	14
9. Ky	(11)	8^13	15	15	12	15	15	15	15	15	15	15	12	15	15	15	6	15
10. Cb	7	12	12	15	12	15	13	15	13	15	15	15	11	15	15	15	15	14
MODALITY	VRB	GST	GST	VRB	GST	GST	GST	GST	VRB	GST	GST	VRB	GPH	GPH	GPH	GPH	GPH	GPH
MINUTES	3	3	2	2	2	1	3	1	2	1	2	3	3	2	2	3	2	3
MEAN SCORE	8.7	11.0	11.6	13.2	12.9	15.0	14.0	15.0	13.5	14.8	15.0	15.0	7.0	14.3	14.5	15.0	13.4	14.3

Response Levels:

Overall 13.23   Gestural 13.46   Verbal 12.60   Graphic 13.08

%ile 84th   %ile 73rd   %ile 59th   %ile 93rd

FIGURE 2–1 Porch Index of Communicative Ability Score Sheet, Modality Response Summary, and Ranked Response Summary for patient S. Dr. B. Porch, *Porch index of communicative ability.* Palo Alto, Calif.: Consulting Psychologists Press, 1967, 1971. Reprinted by permission.

ties. The subtest means also provide information regarding S.'s performance on specific test battery tasks. S. performed substantially poorer on a task which required written descriptions of the functions of objects (Subtest A), for example, than on tasks which required him to write the names of objects presented visually (Subtest B), auditorially (Subtest C), and following oral spelling (Subtest D). Similarly he demonstrated poorer performance on a task requiring him to describe the function of objects (Subtest I) than subtests that assessed object naming (Subtest IV), sentence completion (Subtest IX), and verbal imitation (Subtest XI). Relatively spared reading ability is reflected in the performance of S. on subtests V and VII.

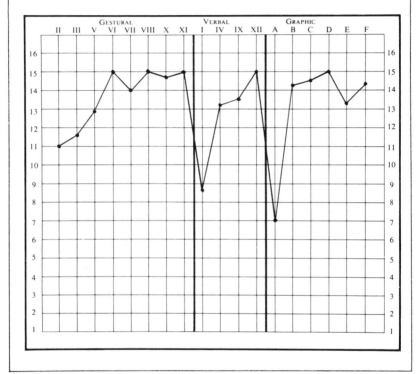

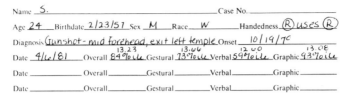

Porch **I**ndex of **C**ommunicative **A**bility

MODALITY RESPONSE SUMMARY

Name _S._ _____ Case No. _____

Age _24_ Birthdate _2/23/57_ Sex _M_ Race _W_ Handedness ⓇⓇ uses Ⓡ

Diagnosis _Gunshot- mid forehead, exit left temple_ Onset _10/19/7__

Date _4/6/81_ Overall _84%ile_ Gestural _73%ile_ Verbal _59%ile_ Graphic _93%ile_
(13.23) (13.66) (12.00) (13.08)

Date _____ Overall _____ Gestural _____ Verbal _____ Graphic _____

Date _____ Overall _____ Gestural _____ Verbal _____ Graphic _____

The modality response summary and the ranked response summary allow examination of S.'s scores as a function of modality and of subtest difficulty respectively. They show the interrelationships of subtest performances and are intended to evaluate change over the course of rehabilitation. If a single statement were used to describe the performance of S. on the PICA, his communication ability would be characterized as adept with little assistance and with relatively better preserved graphic and gestural than verbal output modality functioning.

The performance of S. on the Boston Diagnostic Examination is summa-

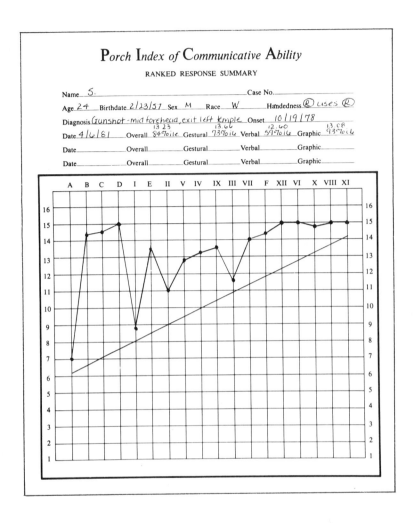

Porch Index of Communicative Ability

RANKED RESPONSE SUMMARY

Name S.   Case No.

Age 24   Birthdate 2/23/57 Sex M   Race W   Handedness ℝ uses ℝ

Diagnosis Gunshot - mid forehead, exit left temple Onset 10/19/78

Date 4/6/81   Overall 84%ile Gestural 73%ile Verbal 59%ile Graphic 93%ile

Date_____Overall_____Gestural_____Verbal_____Graphic_____

Date_____Overall_____Gestural_____Verbal_____Graphic_____

rized in Figure 2–2. Included are a rating scale profile of speech characteristics and a Z score profile of aphasia subscores. The rating scale profile is most consistent with a diagnosis of Broca's aphasia. Aphasia is rated as severe, and conversational speech is marked by poor melody, agrammatism, reduced phrase length, and almost exclusive use of content words. Auditory comprehension is mildly impaired. Differences in S.'s rating configuration compared to a "classic" Broca's aphasic patient are the higher incidence of paraphasia and higher rating of articulatory agility. Examination of the Z score profile also shows a mixed Broca's pattern. Fluency is low compared to relatively spared auditory comprehension. Naming is marginally better than fluency, paraphasias are few, reading is mildly impaired except for oral spelling, and the parietal lobe battery scores are near normal. A marked exception to the expected Broca's pattern is the high writing scores.

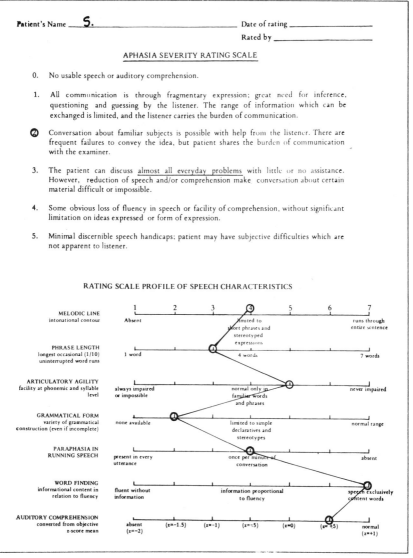

FIGURE 2–2 *Aphasia Severity Rating Scale* and *Z*-Score Profile of Aphasia Subscores for Patient S. From H. Goodglass and E. Kaplan, *Boston Diagnostic Aphasia Examination.* Philadelphia: Lea and Febiger, 1972. Reprinted by permission.

The most logical description of the patient's performance is a moderate mixed Broca's aphasia. Performance on individual tasks of the battery can be evaluated further by comparing S.'s scores on subtests to the performance of the standardization population in *Z* score units (i.e., standard deviations from the mean).

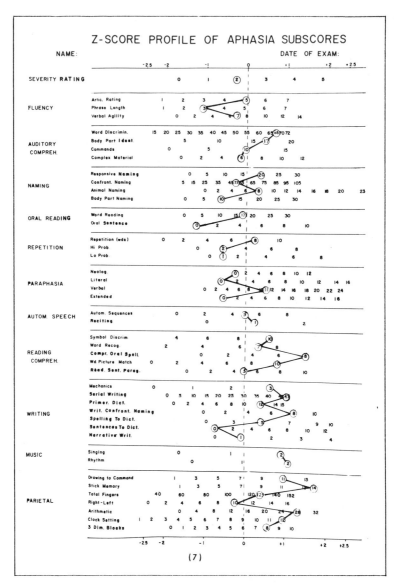

The performance of S. on the functional communication profile is shown in Figure 2–3. It should be remembered that the ratings on the 45 items are based on a premorbid reference—that is, the behaviors rated from direct observation, inference, or report are comparisons to premorbid levels of functioning. The percentiles for S.—Movement, 75 percent; Speaking, 19 percent; Understanding, 70 percent; Reading, 42 percent; and Other, 70 percent—reflect the greater impairment of speaking skills compared to the other areas rated. The overall percentage suggests that his communication effectiveness is 57.4 percent of premorbid level.

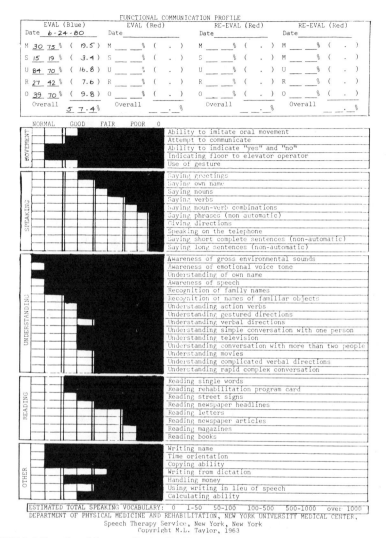

FIGURE 2–3 Functional Communication Profile for patient S. From M. L. Taylor, "A Measurement of Functional Communication in Aphasia," *Archives of Physical Medicine and Rehabilitation* Vol. 46, 101-107, 1963.

Administration of the Communicative Abilities of Daily Living yielded a score of 125 for S. Two comparisons with the standardization population are of interest: S.'s performance compared to aphasic noninstitutionalized males less than 46 years of age and compared to Broca's aphasics as a group. The mean score of the noninstitutionalized males was 111.3 with a standard deviation of 20.4. Therefore, S. scored slightly less than one standard deviation from the mean for this group. The Broca aphasics' mean score was 106.3 with a standard deviation of 22.5. Again, S. scored approximately one standard deviation above the mean. A final interpretive consideration is how closely S.'s score approximates normal functional communication. The cutoff score established for noninstitutionalized males of his age group is 128. A score of 125 can be interpreted to mean that his functional communication ability is near normal.

○ OTHER TESTS FOR NEUROGENIC DISORDERS

While serving as reasonably comprehensive assessment instruments for aphasia and, to a more limited extent, apraxia and dysarthria, aphasia batteries are insufficient for differential diagnosis of other neurogenic disorders. Darley (1979) observed that a ". . . curious failure in aphasia test development relates to the general absence of built-in ways of distinguishing aphasic patients from patients with language disorders that might be confused with aphasia," (p. 192) and "Test makers have not demonstrated that aphasia can be differentiated from syndromes of confusion, dementia, or psychosis through the use of their tests" (p. 192). Other tests must therefore be used that can differentiate disorders that may only resemble aphasia. Additional tests and assessment protocols may be needed to evaluate particular neurogenically based linguistic disorders in more detail. Although not an exhausting list, several tests and test protocols will be reviewed to provide examples of tools available.

The *Token Test* (DeRenzi and Vignolo, 1962) was developed to assess high-level auditory comprehension deficits associated with brain damage. The tokens used are large and small blue, green, red, white, and yellow squares and circles. The patient's task is to manipulate the tokens in response to instructions of increasing length and complexity on the five levels of the test. Initial items include instructions such as "touch the yellow circle," while the more advanced items require the patient to perform tasks such as "put the green square beside the red circle." The test purports to test auditory comprehension, but obviously it also places a considerable burden on memory abilities.

The test has proven useful for testing a wide range of patients including left-brain-damaged with aphasia, brain-damaged without aphasia, and nonbrain-damaged subjects (Orgass and Poeck, 1966; Swisher and Sarno, 1969) and patients with cerebral commissurotomy and hemispherectomy (Zaidel, 1977). A short form of the test is also available (Spellacy and Spreen, 1969).

The *Revised Token Test** (McNeil and Prescott, 1978) is the result of a major effort to standardize the original test which had undergone numerous modifications. Standardization included:

*M. McNeil and T. Prescott, *Revised Token Test.* Baltimore: University Park Press, 1978. Reprinted by permission.

(1) a pretest designed to assess the subject's basic knowledge of colors, shapes, and sizes as well as balanced representation for each;

(2) specific colors (shades), materials and sizes of the tokens;

(3) specific placement of the tokens (designed to reduce the visual search aspect of the subject's performance);

(4) a consistent order of presentation for each subtest and commands within subtests;

(5) a procedure for scoring each linguistic element, each stimulus, each subtest and an overall test mean; and

(6) specific rules for applying each of the fifteen categories in the evaluative system. (p. 20)

The Revised Token Test contains ten subtests and responses are scored by means of a 15-point multidimensional scoring system similar to the one used in the Porch Index of Communicative Ability. The test was standardized on 90 neurologically normal, 30 left-brain-damaged, and 30 right-brain-damaged adults. Percentiles for overall, subtest, and linguistic element means are provided for the three subject groups of the sample. The authors noted that the test appears to be a sensitive instrument for detecting brain damage and the severity levels obtained are efficient at differentiating between auditory comprehension performance in normal, right-brain-damaged, and left-brain-damaged patients.

The *Wechsler Memory Scale* (Wechsler and Stone, 1948) was developed to assess various aspects of visual and auditory memory. The seven subtests include personal and current information (How old are you?); general orientation (What year is this?); mental control (say the letters of the alphabet); logical memory (recall of ideas from two short paragraphs presented auditorily); digits forward and backward (recall of digit series of increasing length); visual reproduction (recall of geometric designs presented for ten seconds); and associative learning (recall of the second word of word pairs presented over three trials). The patient's subtest scores are added, corrected for age, and used to determine an equivalent mental quotient.

The scale was standardized on more than 200 normal adult men and women between 25 and 50 years of age. A score correction for age is provided for patients from 20 to 64 years of age at five-year intervals. The scale requires relatively intact receptive and expressive skills and, therefore, is probably more appropriate for patients with right brain damage, confusion, or dementia than for patients with aphasia.

The *Raven Progressive Matrices* is a nonverbal test which determines intellectual functioning by means of a single factor—visual perception. It is a

test of the ability to apprehend meaningless figures presented for observation, see the relations between them, conceive the nature of the figure completing each system of relations presented, and by doing so, develop a systematic method of reasoning. (Raven, 1960)

The *Standard Progressive Matrices* (Raven, 1960) are composed of 60 items divided into five sets (A, B, C, D, E) of 12 each. On each set the problems become more difficult. Stimuli are black and white drawings from which a part has been removed, and six possible choices are provided to complete the design. The patient chooses which of the foils successfully completes the design. The test is typically untimed and can be individually or group administered. It was designed for children from 6 to 13½ years of age, although the test may be administered at any age; the same items are administered no matter what the age of the patient.

The test was standardized on subjects from 6 to 65 years of age. The score is the total number of right responses which can be compared to percentiles of the normative population, including children and adults. By definition, the test requires intact visual perceptual skills for successful completion.

The *Coloured Progressive Matrices* (Raven, 1963) were designed for children from ages 5 to 11, for elderly people, and for communication-impaired, intellectually subnormal, and intellectually deteriorated patients. It is composed of three sets of 12 items. Sets A and B are identical to the first two sets of the Standard Matrices except they are colored. Test Ab is a new set. The score is the total number correct which can be compared to percentile norms for children and healthy elderly people from 65 to 85 years of age. If the Coloured Matrices are found to be too easy, Sets C, D, and E are administered. The results of Set Ab are then discarded, and the total score is compared to norms for the Standard Matrices.

The Reading Comprehension Battery of Aphasia (RCBA) (LaPointe and Horner, 1979) was developed as a comprehensive reading assessment instrument for aphasic adults but could also be used to focus treatment on the impairment identified. LaPointe and Horner noted that the reading subtests of aphasia batteries were too limited in scope to allow more than a cursory evaluation of the type and severity of reading deficits. They also noted that the content of reading instruments for developmental alexia and reading emergence in school children was often not suitable for adults. The RCBA contains ten subtests each with ten items. Tests range from single-word comprehension and functional reading to sentence and paragraph comprehension and morpho-syntactic reading with lexical controls. Development of the subtests took into consideration such variables as form class, frequency of occurrence, word length, concreteness, imageability, and the nature of the foils used. Each item is scored as pass or fail, and the time for completion of each subtest is recorded. PICA scoring may be used if decided upon by the examiner. All items are to be attempted since no basals or ceilings for performance have been established. Reliability and validity have not been determined since the battery currently is undergoing standardization.

Test results may be used to determine both quantitative and qualitative aspects of the patient's performance. Comparisons of overall, subtest, and items within subtests performance provides quantitative information that can be used to determine whether a disorder exists and to serve as a baseline for determining the effects of therapeutic intervention. As to qualitative judgments, LaPointe and Horner noted that ". . . an individual profile analysis with respect to the various linguistic levels and types of tasks on the RCBA may provide insight as to the level of breakdown and the interrelation between the visual, auditory, semantic, lexical, and morpho-syntactic factors affecting factual, inferential, and functional reading comprehension."

Although only four tests used to aid in appraising neurogenic linguistic disorders have been reviewed, there are many others. For example, the *Peabody Picture Vocabulary Test* (Dunn, 1965), *Gates Advanced Primary Reading Test* (Gates, 1958), *Benton Visual Retention Test* (Benton, 1974), *Templin-Darley Tests of Articulation* (1969), and the *Word Fluency Measure* (Borkowski, Benton, and Spreen, 1969). These tests are selected for administration in order to expand the range of testing for particular linguistic and cognitive deficits insufficiently explored by aphasia batteries or to appraise areas of dysfunction not included on the batteries. Additionally, acquisition of a speech sample analyzed to provide quantitative data on disturbed speech dimensions in dysarthria (Darley, et. al., 1975) or language performance deficits in aphasia (Yorkston and Beukelman, 1980; Chapey, 1981) are of significant value to differential diagnosis and therapy planning. The initial statement of this section must be reemphasized: There are no tests specifically constructed to investigate communicative deficits associated with dementia, confusion, or psychoses. Therefore existent diagnostic materials created for evaluating aphasia and related disorders may need to be employed.

○ PROCEDURES FOR ASSESSING NEUROMOTOR DISORDERS

Acquired neuromotor disorders have been assessed by a number of less formalized procedures, generally outgrowths or modifications of the neurological examination. DeRenzi, Pieczuro, and Vignolo (1966) developed procedures to evaluate oral and limb apraxia. The test included ten oral and ten limb items in which the patients were asked to perform gestures following verbal commands and, if necessary, on imitation. Oral gestures included tasks such as "stick out your tongue," "whistle," and "show how you would kiss someone." Limb gestures included tasks such as "snap your fingers," "make the letter *O* with your finger," and "wave goodbye." Five categories of response were determined; each response was scored as two (correct), one (accurate performance preceded by pause or acceptable performance with defective movements), or zero (important part of gesture absent, perseveration of preceding item, incorrect oral performance, no response). Determination of the presence and severity of oral and limb apraxia was based on the performance of 40 subjects without neurological damage, 40 patients with lesions of the right hemisphere, and 134 patients with damage of the left hemisphere. None of the normal or right-brain-damaged subjects received a score of less than 16 on either the oral or limb tests. Therefore 16 was used as the cutoff point—that is, patients with scores of 15 or less were classified as apractic. The cutoff score for separating mild and severe involvement was set at 11.

Darley et al. (1975) modified the oral apraxia portion of the test by increasing the number of items to 20 and providing 11 categories for grading the response. They also presented 18 test words and phrases useful for eliciting verbal apractic errors such as "gingerbread," "statistical analysis," and "zip-zipper-zippering." Rosenbek and Wertz (1976) expanded the battery of items and integrated verbal, oral, and limb tasks into a single measure. The verbal portion requires the patient to prolong vowels, imitate syllable sequences, and produce words and phrases. Responses are transcribed, scored, and analyzed to determine the type and frequency of phonemic and prosodic errors. The oral apraxia section is identical to the 20 items of Darley et al. (1975), and the limb apraxia test is a modification of the DeRenzi et al. (1966) test. The oral and limb apraxia responses are graded on an 11-point system similar to Darley et al. What has evolved then is a clinical battery offering a comprehensive series of items for evaluating apraxia. The reliability of the battery is unknown, although it would appear to have face validity.

The oral peripheral examination is used to evaluate the functional and anatomic integrity of the speech output system. Included are an assessment of cranial nerves subserving the communication process.

Oral-Peripheral Examination   The oral-peripheral examination is similar to the cranial nerve (CN) examination performed by the physician. The framework for the CN examination is to test functions known to be mediated by each of the nerves. Based on test findings, a decision is made as to whether there is damage to the peripheral nerve or to the structures of the neuroaxis to which it is functionally linked. The oral-peripheral examination differs slightly from the CN examination. Nerves directly involved in the communicative process are tested in detail; nerves subserving other motor and sensory activities are screened or not tested.

Olfaction (CN I) is not typically tested as part of the oral-peripheral examination unless the patient demonstrates dysphagia. Pungent odors stimulate salivation and reflexive swallowing and olfaction is importantly related to the sense of taste. The olfactory nerve is tested by asking the patient to identify a series of substances (oil of cloves, coffee, etc.) presented to each nostril in turn.

The optic nerve (CN II) is assessed because of the high frequency of visual field deficits associated with brain damage. Informal testing is performed by the examiner who, positioned directly behind the patient, randomly and repeatedly introduces a stimulus (finger, pencil, etc.) into the quadrants of the visual field. The patient indicates when he sees the stimulus. Presence of homonymous hemianopsia (loss of vision in half of the visual field) is found contralateral to the damaged hemisphere. Other types of visual field deficits may be identified depending on the site of lesion in the visual pathways.

The oculomotor (CN III), trochlear (CN IV), and abducents (CN VI) motor nerves are not routinely tested. Difficulties in eye movement, ptosis of the eyelid, and deviation of the eye are recorded, however, since they, like visual field deficits, effect the ability of the patient to respond to visual stimuli.

The trigeminal nerve (CN VI) has both sensory and motor fibers. Facial sensation and masticatory muscle function are the primary areas assessed. Informal testing of sensation is carried out by requiring the patient, who has his eyes closed, to point to the area of the face stroked with a piece of cotton. Jaw muscles are tested by palpating the masseter and temporalis while the teeth are clenched, examining the jaw at rest for deviation, and requiring the patient to open and close the jaw against an applied resistance.

The facial nerve (CN VII) also has sensory and motor fibers. Taste to the anterior two-thirds of the tongue is not tested except if the patient demonstrates dysphagia. The face is examined at rest and during lip spreading and rounding for signs of weakness. Strength is also evaluated by asking the patient to move the lips against an applied resistance.

Testing of the auditory nerve (CN VIII) is not routinely completed in the oral-peripheral examination. Auditory testing including pure tone, speech reception, and speech discrimination tests are completed as part of the comprehensive assessment of the patient.

The glossopharyngeal (CN IX), vagus (CN X), and accessory (CN XI) nerves contain both sensory and motor fibers and are tested together insofar as they innervate the palatopharyngeal and laryngeal musculature. The soft palate is examined at rest to determine if it deviates towards one side and during phonation and elicitation of a gag reflex to evaluate faucial pillar and palatal movement. Nasality is judged during phonation with the nostrils open and occluded. Voice quality, pitch, and loudness during phonation and speech tasks are used to assess laryngeal function.

Tongue musculature is innervated by the hypoglossal (CN XII) nerve. Evaluative tasks include examination of the tongue at rest and during protrusion, circular, and back and forth movements. The patient is also asked to move the tongue against an applied resistance on the left and right sides in turn.

In addition to the tasks briefly described above, structures (face, tongue, teeth, alveolar ridge, hard palate, soft palate) are examined for size, shape, symmetry, structural abnormalities, and relationship to one another. Diadochokinetic rates are also established for nonverbal lip, jaw, and tongue movements and for individual and combined bilabial, lingua-dental, and linguavelar syllables.

Finally, other assessment procedures have been developed which might better be termed protocols than tests. Larsen (1972) described a protocol for evaluating swallowing dysfunction (dysphagia) due to neuromuscular disorders. Included within the evaluation are a history (patient complaint, eating habits, foods preferred, incidence of choking); examination of the speech mechanism (muscle strength and structural range of motion); evaluation of swallowing (volitional and reflexive); determination of the integrity of taste sensation (sweet, sour, salty); and ability of the patient to masticate and swallow various nutritional substances (liquids, solids, dry, moist). A similar protocol was developed for deglutition deficits by Bell and Goepfert (1977).

○ EXAMINER AND PATIENT VARIABILITY

If reliable and valid estimates of the patient's deficits and residual capacities are to be made, the communicative and personal interaction between the patient and the examiner within the test situation must be considered. In general the examiner's skills and experience are more important than the tests selected to assess the communicative deficits, and the patient's physical and emotional status are critical determiners of his or her responses.

Examiner Effects The attitude of the examiner is important. Stoicheff (1960) investigated the speech behavior of 42 aphasic patients under three types of motivating instructions: encouraging, discouraging, and nonevaluative. She found that the patients performed more poorly on reading and naming tasks and rated themselves as performing more poorly under the discouraging compared to the encouraging condition. The implication is that the anxiety of the patient is strongly influenced by the attitude of the examiner and may have important effects on task performance.

A second examiner effect derives from alterations to test item procedures. Some tests, notably the Porch Index of Communicative Ability, specify with great care how items are to be administered. Other tests are much more flexible in terms of administration, scoring of responses, and reinforcement. The effects of these alterations can only be determined by the examiner.

Patient Effects Quite obviously the level of consciousness of the patient is important. Four levels are generally recognized: alertness, lethargy or somnolence, stupor or semicoma, and coma (Strub and Black, 1977). The alert patient is able to interact meaningfully with the examiner.

The arousal state is required for the establishment of vigilance (ability to maintain attention for an extended period of time). The lethargic patient is not fully alert and drifts off to sleep if not specifically stimulated. Such patients cannot maintain attention, and their awareness of the immediate surroundings is limited. *Stupor* and *semicoma* are terms used to describe patients who can only be aroused by vigorous and persistent stimulation. The patient at this level of consciousness does not arouse spontaneously, and no meaningful assessment of communicative functioning can be conducted. The comatose patient does not respond to either external or internal stimuli, and the term *coma* is reserved for patients at the bottom of the scale of consciousness or arousability. Only patients who are fully alert and attentive should be administered test batteries since the tests are premised on the assumption that a maximal performance of the patient has been achieved.

Fatigue may affect test results. Patients who have recently incurred brain damage tire easily and may find the testing situation demanding of their energies. Testing may have to be divided into several short sessions to counteract the negative effects of fatigue. Since the typical neurologically involved patient is elderly, visual and auditory sensory deficits resulting from or coexistent with brain damage may affect responses. Procedures and materials may need to be altered or modified to maximize the performance of the patient.

Finally, the emotional status of the patient is important. Brain-damaged patients frequently find testing to be anxiety producing. They may be depressed from loss of physical and communicative functioning and find the hospital or rehabilitation facility inhospitable and threatening. They may find their inability to perform frustrating and new situations overwhelming in terms of the magnitude of environmental stimuli that must be dealt with.

○ CONTEXT

In differential diagnosis of communication disorders, test results provide only a part of the information that will be needed from the client. Social, familial, educational, and medical information provide the factual background needed to put the results of the testing into perspective (Table 2–5). To a large extent, the amount of contextual information available when the patient is assessed is dependent on the environment where the speech-language pathologist works. The hospital environment usually includes a large number of professionals directly involved with the care of the patient and therefore provides a large body of integrated factual data. If the patient has been discharged, the information may be available but will typically be summarized as a discharge report. If at all possible, information should be obtained from all hospitals, rehabilitation facilities, and private

TABLE 2–5

A. *Identifying Information:* Name, age, sex, birthdate, address, clinic number, physician, telephone number.

B. *Pre-Onset of Brain Damage Information:*
   1. *Educational History:* Years of education and schools attended; academic performance.
   2. *Vocational History:* Type, place, and length of employment; family income.
   3. *Family Structure:* Marital status, number of children and ages, living environment.
   4. *Personality and Interests:* Personality characteristics (cheerfulness, motivation, aggressiveness, cooperativeness); interests, recreational pursuits, hobbies.
   5. *Medical History:* Incidences of brain damage, confusion, disorientation, metabolic disturbances, hypertension, or other medical problems; where treated and by whom; names, addresses, and specialities of physicians.
   6. *Handedness:* Left, right, ambidextrous.
   7. *Speech/Language History:* Articulation deficits, stuttering, hearing loss; Where, when, and by whom treated.

C. *Post-Onset of Brain Damage Information:*
   1. Where onset occurred, symptoms, hospital or physician where patient conveyed, attending physician, treatment administered.
   2. Results of medical/neurological examination:
      a. Mental status: memory, speech and language functioning, alertness, orientation, etc.
      b. Cranial nerve results.
      c. Sensory and motor deficits.
      d. Other medical findings.
      e. Initial diagnosis of type, location, and size of lesion.
   3. Tests ordered and results: electroencepholography, computerized axial tomography, angiography, etc.
   4. Medications ordered and dosages.
   5. Referrals to other rehabilitation specialities and results of their examinations. Type and intensity of treatment if already initiated.
   6. Mental status since admission: alertness, orientation, motivation, etc.

practitioners since the patient or another member of the family who serves as the informant may not be fully aware of the type, extent, and size of the neurological lesion and the course of treatment or prognosis.

The first step in establishing contextual information is to obtain the patient's personal history, including social, educational, and vocational background. Questions of importance will include the patient's age, sex, family structure (marital status, number of children), education, place and type of employment, living environment, income, hobbies, and personality characteristics. The purpose of this information gathering is to gain as complete a picture as possible of the patient as a person up to the moment of testing. A standard case history form is typically utilized for this purpose because it provides structure for the interviewing process. Case history forms and procedures are available elsewhere (Darley and Spriestersbach, 1978).

Medical history should be obtained from the patient's chart if he or she is hospitalized or in the form of a medical summary if he or she is not. Information from the records will typically include reports of past illnesses and trauma, the results of medical and neurological examinations, the reports of laboratory tests, nurses' and doctors' notes, and the treatment and course of recovery.

The medical history should be reviewed carefully for information regarding earlier incidences of brain damage, periods of confusion or disorientation, and complicating conditions such as metabolic diseases, cardiac disease, or seizure. The results of the neurological examination provide data on the site, size, and nature of the lesion and possible progression of the disorder. The neurological examination performed by the physician specifically includes the evaluation of mental state, cranial nerve function, motor and reflex systems, the cerebellar apparatus, sensory modalities, and the autonomic nervous system. Evaluation of mental state includes assessment of intellectual facility and fund of knowledge; orientation for time, place, and person; memory; attention span; understanding of simple and complex commands; general information; calculation; and abstract thinking and judgment (Alpers and Mancall, 1971). More recently Strub and Black (1977) have advocated the use of portions of psychometric batteries as part of the process for determining the mental status of the patient.

The cranial nerves are assessed by testing the sensory and motor functions of the areas of the body that they subserve. Examination of the motor systems provides information on muscle power, bulk, and tone; active and passive movements; involuntary movements; cerebellar functioning, and status of the reflexes. Evaluation of sensory function includes investigation of touch, pain, heat, cold, position, vibration, and a variety of discriminatory senses. An attempt is made to determine what elements of sensation are affected, the degree of involvement, and the areas of sensory impairment or loss.

Laboratory tests are an important part of the process for establishing the type and extent of brain damage and have been described by Alpers and Mancall (1971). *Electroencephalography* involves recording the electrical activity generated by the cortex in order to isolate areas of abnormal rhythm or amplitude which are generated by focal lesions. *Angiography* is a technique in which a radioactive substance is introduced into an artery subserving the brain. Subsequent skull X-rays allow a determination of structural abnormalities of blood vessels caused by vascular malformations and aneurysms and the presence of stenotic and thrombosed vessels or neoplasms. The X-rays also reveal alterations in the position of vessels caused by mass lesions and alterations in flow patterns caused by circulatory malformations and tumors.

Pneumoencephalography entails the introduction of air into the ventricular system followed by contrast radiography. It is of particular value in identifying cerebral atrophy, hydrocephalus, and neoplasms. Atrophy and hydrocephalus are evidenced by a marked enlargement of the ventricles, and a space-occupying lesion is indicated by a distortion in the size and shape of the ventricles. Strokes, tumors, abscesses, and hematomas can also be located by means of a *brain scan*. The technique involves the injection of a radioactive fluid into an artery leading to the brain. The brain is then scanned for concentrations of radioactivity. Increased concentrations of blood are seen as darker areas that indicate possible sites of lesion. *Computerized transaxial tomography* is another radiographic technique. Based upon computer-processed data derived from "slices" through the cranium, both normal and pathological structures can be identified. This technique to a large extent has replaced some of the procedures described earlier because it can be used to evaluate the entire cerebrum with almost no risk to the patient. In isolated instances, however, the results of the scan may be supplemented by results from other tests.

Based upon medical history, physical examination, and the results of laboratory tests, an estimate of the site, size, and nature of the lesion and whether it is a static or progressive condition are determined and recorded in the medical records. This information is critical to the differential diagnosis process since the status of the brain is the most potent determinant of the type of communication problem demonstrated by the patient.

The nurses' notes offer information of the alertness of the patient: his orientation to time, place, and person and his adjustment to the problem. The physical status of the patient, results of recent laboratory findings, ordered medications, and prescribed course of treatment are included in the doctors' notes.

The results of a clinician's testing, then, are combined with the personal history, medical history, results of the neurological examination and laboratory tests, and the observations of other health workers charged with the care of the patient. The patient may be evaluated when only a portion of this information is available, but a clinician's ability to make decisions regarding diagnosis and prognosis will be significantly enhanced by the acquisition of these data.

○ DIFFERENTIAL DIAGNOSIS

Differential diagnosis is the process of assigning a label to the behavioral characteristics of a particular communicative disorder. From the tests reviewed this might appear to be a simplistic task since the assessment results offer a sufficient number of behavioral observations to allow dichotomous decisions to facilitate the labeling process. This is hardly the case. The diagnostic process is rendered difficult by two features of communicative disorders associated with brain damage. First, deficits are not limited to any particular disorder. Comparison of the performance of patients with aphasia, apraxia, generalized intellectual impairment, and confusion (Halpern, et al., 1973) with that of schizophrenic patients (DiSimoni, Darley, and

Aronson, 1977) revealed deficits in common for the five groups. Results from patient performance on ten tasks (auditory retention, adequacy, arithmetic, auditory comprehension, fluency, naming, syntax, reading comprehension, writing, and relevance) revealed that all five groups were impaired on at least seven of the tasks. Even though five of the tasks were helpful in differentiating the groups, the overlap of communicative deficits suggests that the presence of a deficit, or even a group of deficits, may not allow reliable differential diagnosis.

A second related problem is that neurogenic communicative disorders seldom occur in isolation. For example, Wertz, Rosenbek and Deal (1970) investigated the incidence of disorders coexistent with apraxia. They found that 65 percent of the patients demonstrated apraxia of speech with aphasia, 14 percent displayed apraxia with aphasia and dysarthria, 13 percent had apraxia only, and 8 percent showed apraxia and dysarthria. The difficulties in drawing diagnostic lines between disorders is no mean task for even the experienced examiner. These difficulties are complicated further because little information is available on communicative disabilities associated with confusion and dementia and few speech-language pathologists have extensive experience working with these patients. The lack of experience may be because physicians historically have not referred patients who demonstrate communicative disorders that are transient, such as in acute confusional states, or that have poor prognoses for recovery, such as dementia.

The task here is to provide a very brief framework for differential diagnosis. To accomplish this goal, the appraisal tools for each of five diagnostic categories (aphasia, apraxia, dysarthria, general intellectual deterioration, and the language of confusion) will be provided, and the primary characteristics that allow a differential diagnosis of each of the disorders will be considered.

aphasia

Appraisal The tests available to assess aphasia have been reviewed earlier. In general, the Aphasia Language Performance Scales are an excellent screening test. Diagnostic tests of particular merit include the Porch Index of Communicative Ability, the Boston Diagnostic Aphasia Examination, and the Neurosensory Comprehensive Test of Aphasia since they are standardized. Each battery contains tests of auditory comprehension, reading, writing, and oral expression—primary areas to be evaluated in aphasia. Additional measures used may include the Token Test to gain additional information about auditory comprehension, the apraxia battery of Wertz and Rosenbek since aphasics may demonstrate motor performance deficits regardless of site of lesion (Kimura, 1976; Mateer and Kimura, 1977), and a Functional Communication Profile or CADL to gain an estimate of the patients typical performance in everyday settings. Finally, the Raven Coloured Matrices, a speech sample (if not already included in the test battery), and examination of the speech mechanism should be completed.

Diagnosis The typical aphasic patient has suffered an acute onset of symptoms due to rapid occurrence of brain damage. Test results show auditory comprehension, oral expression, and reading and writing deficits although the modalities may not be equally involved. The patient may demonstrate some disorientation for time, place, and person, at least in an acute state, but does not necessarily show paresis, paralysis, or incoordination of the speech production mechanism, with the exception of lower facial weakness contralateral to the damaged hemisphere. Intelligence testing reveals relatively unimpaired intellectual functioning on performance tasks compared to the severe involvement of the patient on verbal tasks.

Aphasia is differentially diagnosed from apraxia on the basis of the relative equity of involvement on language comprehension, oral expression, and reading and writing tasks; from dysarthria by the preservation of neuromuscular innervation to the speech production apparatus as revealed by an oral-peripheral examination; from generalized intellectual impairment on the basis of near-normal performance on nonverbal intelligence measures; and from confusional states by relatively intact orientation and judgment after neurological stability has been reached.

apraxia

Appraisal The question of whether apraxia of speech is a nonlinguistic motor programming disorder or part of a larger language deficit has not been resolved. Consequently assessment should include both language and speech measures. Typical assessment instruments should include an aphasia battery such as the Porch Index of Communicative Abilities or the Boston Diagnostic Aphasia Examination, oral-peripheral examination of the speech mechanism, an apraxia battery (Rosenbek and Wertz, 1976), a speech sample, and an articulation test.

Diagnosis The typical apractic patient has suffered rapid onset, focal brain damage to the left anterior dominant hemisphere. He is younger than the typical aphasic patient (Obler, Albert, Goodglass, and Benson, 1978) and more frequently has an associated hemiplegia contralateral to the damaged hemisphere. Apraxia is differentiated from aphasia on the basis of relatively normal auditory comprehension compared to oral expression; from the language of confusion and generalized intellectual deterioration on the basis of more intact orientation, memory, and learning abilities; and from dysarthria by the preponderance of phonemic substitutions compared to distortion errors (Johns and Darley, 1970), intact neuromuscular functioning with the exception of facial weakness, and hemiplegia.

dysarthria

Appraisal The dysarthric patient is not expected to have marked language, intellectual, cognitive, memory, or learning deficits unless they are associated with the disease process that produced the dysarthria. The primary differential diagnosis to be made is between dysarthria and apraxia. Appraisal instruments include a speech sample, oral-peripheral examination of the speech mechanism, and articulation testing.

Diagnosis The variety of diseases that produce dysarthria makes it difficult to present a typical patient. He may be young or old; the neurological lesion may be large or small, focal or diffuse; the lesion may be anywhere in the motor pathways from the cortex to the muscle fibers. Key characteristics that differentiate dysarthria from apraxia are a preponderance of distortion, rather than substitution, phonemic errors and the presence of neuromuscular involvement of the speech production apparatus as the primary etiology of the communication disorder.

confusion and dementia

Appraisal Both confusion and dementia arise from bilateral hemispheric involvement. The etiology of confusion typically entails an acute reversible systemic dysfunction causing a transient alteration in cerebral activity. Dementia, however, is an insidious irreversible disorder closely associated with the aging process. The appraisal tools for both disorders will include an oral-peripheral examination, memory and orientation tasks from the Wechsler Memory Scale, administration of an aphasia battery, and intelligence testing.

Diagnosis The disorders are differentiated from aphasia on the basis of relatively intact vocabulary, fluency, and reading comprehension. Moreover, the patient with dementia demonstrates higher verbal than performance intelligence quotients while the aphasic patient does better on performance intelligence tasks. Confusion is differentiated from dementia by the rapid onset and variable course of the disorder and by the confabulated responses of the confused patient; dementia is characterized by the patient's exhibiting greater long-term difficulty than the confused patient on complex reading and writing tasks.

○ CLINICAL EXAMPLES

It is customary to present classic cases of specific disorders—either to point out their characteristics or to note the pattern of their test results. In a more realistic sense, few patients fit well into the categories that clinicians sometimes dictate they should, and it is a misrepresentation of standard clinical operations to imply that they do. On the other hand, providing some examples of test instruments used to assess the communicative disorders of neurogenic patients would appear to be a worthwhile endeavor. Five reasonably consecutive referrals to a rehabilitation center and the tests used to appraise the patients' disorders will be reviewed with this purpose in mind. The primary instruments of appraisal selected will be emphasized rather than the more informal observations and analyses of communicative functioning.

Patient J., a 63-year-old vocational counselor, was referred four months following a small left occipital lobe cerebrovascular accident. A neuropsychological examination, including administration of the Wechsler Adult Intelligence Scale (WAIS) and Halstead Reitan Battery, was completed prior to referral. Results of the WAIS yielded a verbal intelligence quotient of 100, a performance quotient of 71, and a full scale score of 87. The Halstead Reitan Battery showed deficits in memory and cognitive functioning, a right visual field deficit, alexia, and constructional apraxia. The tentative diagnosis established was alexia without agraphia and a generalized organic deterioration in intellectual functioning. Speech and language assessment was intended to document and evaluate in greater detail the characteristics of the communicative impairment. Instruments selected included a case history, Boston Diagnostic Aphasia Examination, Mental Status Questionnaire (Goldfarb, 1975), and oral-peripheral examination including visual field testing. On the case history J. demonstrated difficulty in computing her age and in recalling events following the stroke. On the Mental Status Questionnaire she could not remember the date, month of the year, or current or previous president of the United States which suggested a moderate organic brain syndrome. The Boston Aphasia Test revealed normal fluency, repetition, automatic speech, and musical abilities. However J. demonstrated marked difficulty on word discrimination items requiring identification of pictures of objects, letters, forms, actions, colors, and numbers but not on auditory comprehension subtests that included body part identification, right-left discrimination, or ability to follow commands. Responses to auditorily presented complex ideas were correct. Responsive naming was not impaired, but significant deficits were found in confrontation naming in response to visually presented stimuli and in animal and body-part naming. J. could not orally read words or sentences, comprehend items involving symbol discrimination, match words to pictures or read sentences and paragraphs. She could write without difficulty but could not read what she had written. She could not perform written confrontation naming. Oral-peripheral examination of the speech mechanism was unremarkable. Visual field testing revealed a right hemonymous homianopsia. These findings are consistent with a diagnosis of alexia secondary to left occipital lobe cerebrovascular accident complicated by behavioral manifestations of dementia.

Seveal aspects of J's evaluation bear comment. First, neuropsychological data bearing on the communicative impairment was available upon referral and served to guide the selection of assessment measures. It is uncommon to encounter a patient in a hospital or rehabilitation center who has not received at least a mental status screening examination to isolate the general nature of the problem and guide test selection. Second, the information from both the neuropsychological and speech-language evaluations were integral, in this case, to establishing the diagnosis. The WAIS results at first appeared incongruous—it is expected that the effect of a dominant hemisphere lesion would yield a reduced verbal, compared to performance, intelligence quotient. However since dementia typically produces reduced performance compared to verbal scores and the lesion was only proximal to the classical speech and language representational areas, the findings are not paradoxical. The results of the WAIS, Mental Status Questionnaire, case history, and Halstead Reitan test are indicative of dementia. The performance on the Boston test—intact speech and language skills with the exception of a marked deficit in processing visual stimuli—provide documentation of symptoms best termed alexia.

Patient B., a 16-year-old high school student, suffered a stab wound to the left parietal-occipital area which resulted in an infected hematoma requiring craniotomy. At the time of testing he was neurologically stable. Instruments and procedures used included case history, auditory and visual testing, the Boston Diagnostic Aphasia Examination, Token Test, and Reading Comprehension Battery for Aphasia. Examination of the speech mechanism was unremarkable, visual field testing revealed a right visual field deficit, and thresholds obtained by pure-tone audiometric screening were within normal limits bilaterally. Results of the Boston Examination were consistent with an anomic aphasia characterized by mild naming problems, reduced reading comprehension, and auditory comprehension deficits. The Reading Battery results showed correct, albeit delayed, responses to at least 9 of the 10 items on each subtest with the exception of the functional reading subtest where a moderate deficit was identified. Near-normal results were obtained on the Token Test with difficulty noted only on Subtests IV and V which include longer and more complex items. The diagnosis, then, was mild anomic aphasia with an associated right visual field deficit. The rationale for test selection was to assess communicative functioning in a comprehensive fashion and then to do more extensive testing of identified reading and auditory comprehension deficits.

Patient P., a 34-year-old woman, was referred with a history of stroke syndrome secondary to strep meningitis involving the entire left hemisphere. She had severe aphasia, right hemiplegia, and right homonymous hemianopsia. Tests administered included the Aphasia Language Performance Scales (ALPS), Minnesota Test for the Differential Diagnosis of Aphasia (MTDDA), and Communicative Abilities of Daily Living (CADL).

Additional appraisal procedures included case history, auditory and visual field testing, and examination of the speech mechanism. Results of the ALPS showed severe involvement of listening, talking, and writing skills and a profound deficit in reading. Administration of the MTDDA indicated profoundly reduced functioning in all modalities most consistent with assignment of the patient to Group V—irreversible aphasia syndrome. A score of 41 was obtained on the CADL which was more than 50 points below the most severely involved noninstitutionalized female patient of the standardization population. A mild right facial weakness and right visual field deficit were shown by the oral-peripheral examination which included visual field testing. These findings are consistent with a diagnosis of severe aphasia with associated visual field deficit. Functional communication is marginal and prognosis for recovery poor.

Patient C., a 49-year-old male, was referred following a bilateral brainstem infarct with resultant quadriplegia and dysarthria. Appraisal procedures included case history, oral-peripheral examination, acquisition of a speech sample, recording of a standard reading passage, and auditory testing. The oral-peripheral examination revealed bilateral facial and velopharyngeal weakness, and weakness of the left side of the tongue. Diadochokinetic rates, intelligibility of conversational speech, and intensity and frequency ranges were moderately reduced. Voice quality was breathy. A moderate bilateral sensorineural hearing loss was shown by audiological assessment. No cognitive or language deficits were reported by the patient or demonstrated from mental status examination. Since there was no indication of hemispheric brain damage and the primary muscular deficit was weakness, the diagnosis was moderate flaccid dysarthria secondary to brainstem infarct.

Patient S., a 62-year-old college professor, was referred with a four-year history of Parkinson's disease characterized by resting tremor of the limbs, muscular rigidity, and paucity of movement. Additionally the patient had suffered a mild right cerebrovascular accident three years prior to referral but at the time of testing did not have any significant residual effects. Appraisal procedures included oral-peripheral examination, recording of a speech sample and standard reading passage, and auditory testing. The oral-peripheral examination revealed tremor of the tongue at rest, restricted lingual range of motion, and higher diadochokinetic rates than normal, but irregular in rhythm. Monotonous pitch, variations in speaking rate, prolongation and repetition of initial sounds and syllables, and mildly reduced intelligibility were noted during conversational speech and to a lesser extent during the reading passage. Auditory acuity was within normal limits bilaterally. The diagnosis was moderate hypokinetic dysarthria secondary to Parkinson's disease.

Two final points need to be made about these examples. First, the tests cited were not the only appraisal tools used over the course of rehabilitation.

The intent was to select those that would effectively allow differential diagnosis of the type and severity of the disorder. Additional measures were employed to evaluate, for example, articulatory skills in the dysarthric patients and grammatical skills in the aphasic patients. They were administered at a later point to more effectively plan the therapy regime. Seldom are the procedures used to determine the diagnosis sufficient alone to quantify the communication deficits to be addressed in treatment. Secondly, the standardized tests could have been replaced by others. For example, the Boston test could have been replaced by the PICA without significant effects on the ability to isolate the communicative deficits. No standardized test battery is ever mandatory to the evaluation of the patient.

Identification of acquired neurogenic communication disorders requires the use of calibrated assessment instruments, the gathering of contextual biographical and medical information, and the assignment of a label to the disorder based upon test findings and contextual information. It is of utmost importance to rehabilitation because information obtained during the identification process also serves as part of the data base for determining a prognosis for recovery and for describing in quantifiable terms the communication deficits that will need to be addressed in the rehabilitation process.

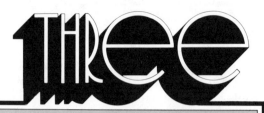

Prognosis

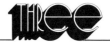

○ INTRODUCTION

Discussion of the salient characteristics of neurogenic disorders and of appraisal instruments and diagnostic procedures serves as a prelude to discussion of rehabilitation. *Rehabilitation* is defined as a maximizing of residual abilities and best describes the goal of therapeutic intervention strategies for patients with acquired neurogenic communication disorders.

The first topics to be addressed include the physiological bases of recovery, the efficacy of treatment, and prognostic indicators. *Physiological recovery* will be considered because, as a minimum requirement, the rehabilitation procedures implemented must significantly enhance communicative effectiveness beyond that expected from the patient's response to damage. It serves, then, as the reference against which therapeutic gains are to be measured. The *efficacy of treatment,* from an objective standpoint, involves decisions on which procedures are appropriate and beneficial to the patient. If the patient's communicative ability is not significantly improved, or in the case of progressive disorders, the patient's communicative integrity is not maintained over a period of time, then the treatment paradigm cannot withstand the criticism that the clinician's time is wasted and the patient's financial resources misspent. Bound up with the discussion of efficacy is prognosis. *Prognosis* is the prediction of future performance based upon factual indicants of the patient's condition and the expected benefits of treatment. At issue are the effects of the therapy program. A physician does not haphazardly prescribe drugs in varying amounts disregarding the medical condition to be treated. Knowing the diagnosis and the patient, the physician uses drugs with known ameliorative effects at specified dosages to accomplish an intended goal. Likewise, factual indicants of the patient's condition must be considered in deciding on a course of treatment with predictable effects on communicative adequacy. Speech language pathologists can no longer operate on the principle that some treatment is always better than no treatment and that any gain derived from the treatment is sufficient to merit the rehabilitative effort.

○ BASES OF REHABILITATION: PHYSIOLOGICAL RECOVERY, TREATMENT EFFICACY, PROGNOSIS

At 3 A.M. on June 17, 1783, Dr. Samuel Johnson, the famed English lexicographer, awoke to find that he could not speak. He immediately tested his mental faculties by composing a prayer in Latin. Next he tried to loosen his powers of speech by drinking wine, but the wine caused him to go back to sleep. When he awoke, he still could not speak and summoned his physicians. Blisters to each side of the throat, to the head, and to the back were prescribed along with salts of hartshorn, and an excellent prognosis for recovery was predicted. The prognosis was well-founded, and Dr. Johnson's speech began returning in a day or two and continued to improve for the next month. Eventually he was left with only a stable dysarthria.

Several aspects of this description of Dr. Johnson's aphasia by Rosner (1974) merit comment. First, it appears in light of modern medical practice that Dr. Johnson's recovery was due to "spontaneous" physiological restitution since it could not be ascribed to the treatment applied. At the same time it must be assumed that his physicians, who applied a valueless treatment to the wrong part of the body, must have had some reason to believe that the prescribed blisters were the most efficacious treatment known. It cannot be determined what prognostic indicators they employed or the scientific bases for the treatment applied, but it can be assumed that the recovery strengthened their belief in the treatment and the prognostic indicators used. Three aspects of Dr. Johnson's aphasia—physiological recovery, efficacy of treatment, and prognostic indicators—will serve as the launching point for discussion of rehabilitation. These three topics are inexorably bound—the efficacy of treatment cannot be determined without knowledge of expected physiological recovery, and the prognosis cannot be reliably determined without information on the physiological status of the patient and the estimated value of the treatment.

○ PHYSIOLOGICAL BASES OF RECOVERY

The etiologies of brain damage that produce neurogenic communication disorders were briefly discussed in Chapter One. At this point, the physiological processes that underlie the organism's response to a lesion will be described in more detail. The purpose of this discussion is to develop an understanding of the patient's behavioral changes following damage so that the time course of communicative return can be examined more carefully.

physiological processes of normal brain function

Three physiological processes underlying normal brain function are the functionally bonded activity of cerebral blood flow, metabolism, and neurotransmitter substances.

Cerebral Blood Flow Oxygen and glucose are needed for normal brain metabolism. Oxygen is carried in the hemoglobin of red blood cells; glucose is transported in blood serum. Approximately one-third of the blood flow to the brain is through the basilar artery; two-thirds through the carotid system, often slightly more on the left side (Lewis, 1976). The capillary system of white matter is less dense than that of gray matter and is metabolically less active (Bloom and Fawcett, 1975).

Lassen et al. (1978) demonstrated that there is increased blood flow and oxygen usage during mental and physical activity that Roland (1980) ascribed to ". . . tight coupling between neuronal and glial metabolism, glucose consumption, and regional cerebral blood flow" (p. 27). The regulation of blood flow to brain tissue is controlled by mechanisms that respond to changes in cerebral vasculature perfusion pressure and to changes in the oxygen and carbon dioxide content of arterial blood and also by mechanisms that assure an adequate blood supply to brain tissue and that restrict blood inflow through arteries (Mchedlishvili, 1980). Basically, then, the cerebral blood flow regulatory mechanisms insure that glucose and oxygen delivered to brain tissue are sufficient to subserve the functions undertaken as indicated by the activity of neurons.

Metabolism The brain requires a large energy supply provided by oxygen and glucose in order to maintain neuronal membrane potentials and other cellular activities. Despite this large and continuous demand, the brain lacks oxygen stores and has limited glucose reserves (Lewis, 1976; Tower, 1979). If blood flow is disrupted, the brain is unable to utilize derivatives of metabolism as energy sources, and neuronal function is impaired.

Neurotransmitters Neurotransmitters are chemical mediators of impulse transmission at synaptic junctions that serve either excitatory or inhibitory functions. They are present in nerve fibers that innervate cerebral vessels (Edvinsson and Owman, 1979; Lewis, 1976) as well as other neural tissue. It has been suggested that neural control exists for regulation of blood flow (Edvinsson & Owman, 1979) and that much of the energy required by the brain is involved in the synthesis, storage, and re-uptake of these transmitters.

The effect of a brain lesion is a bilateral reduction in hemispheric blood flow, disrupted metabolism, and abnormal release of neurotransmitters. Intracranial pressure is also increased due to edema, tumor growth, or hemorrhagic mass causing distortion, compression, and displacement of the hemispheres. Finally, diaschisis occurs which West (1978) described as "... an hypothesized *passive transient state* of reduced or abolished function, arising immediately after a brain injury and acting on a neural region *remote* from the lesion" (p. 413). Each of these dysfunctions are factors in the physiological recovery of the patient—that is, as these processes gravitate back toward normal levels of operation, improved communicative ability is seen. Since there is some variation in the processes as a function of etiology, the time course of changes will be considered for each type.

physiological recovery processes following brain damage

The impact of a cerebral lesion on communication is determined by the site, size, etiology, and speed of onset. Rubens (1977) described the time course of the physiological response of the organism to brain damage. He noted that following an ischemic stroke there is no swelling or tissue death for the first day. During the second and third days, edema becomes evident and may compress and displace structures at a considerable distance from the site of infarct. By the end of the first week, the swelling has significantly diminished, and the area of dead tissue has been invaded by new capillaries and macrophages (cells responsible for engulfing and dissipating dead tissue). After several months, the infarcted tissue has disappeared, and a cystic cavity is evident.

The time course of physiological changes associated with hemorrhages and tumors described by Rubens do not mirror those of ischemic lesions. Most hemorrhages develop within the context of long-standing arterial hypertension and involve intracerebral arteries within the subcortical gray. Rupture of the artery brings about a rapid formation of a blood mass within the hemisphere. Massive hemorrhages produce high mortality, but more limited occurrences with survival are characterized by a compression of the ipsilateral and, in some cases, the contralateral hemisphere. The hemorrhage may not directly destroy cortical tissue of the representational areas for speech and language but may compress and distort these areas producing aphasia. Rubens (1977) observed that the physiological recovery in hemorrhage may be delayed. At one week post-onset there may be swelling with compression and distortion of the hemispheres, but after six weeks, swelling has resolved. A major source of the delayed recovery appears to be the relatively slow reduction of the hemorrhagic mass.

Tumors produce different effects. They develop from glial cells and separate neural tissue without actually producing neuronal cell loss. Their effects are slow in evolution and do not appear to produce major changes until the mass of the tumor produces intracranial pressure. The symptoms resolve with reduction of the edema and intracerebral pressure when medications are administered.

Coupled to the increase in intracranial pressure and distortion of the cerebral hemispheres are other cerebral dysfunctions associated with acute lesions. In a study of six patients with acute lesions, Hoedt-Rasmussen and Skinhoj (1964) first observed a bilateral reduction in cerebral blood flow. Meyer, Shinohara, Kanda, Fukuuchi, Ericsson, and Kok (1970) observed that 22 patients, studied 3 to 16 days after onset, demonstrated a bilateral depression of hemispheric blood flow that persisted for two to three weeks but which gradually progressed toward normal levels on the healthy side. Blood flow on the diseased hemisphere remained low. Moreover, Meyer et al. found a significant positive correlation between the duration of symptoms in days and differences in blood flow between the two hemispheres. Bilateral reductions in hemispheric blood flow also have been found in patients with unilateral brain tumors (Shenkin, 1961). Meyer et al. (1970) concluded:

> The only logical explanation of the bilateral reduction of HBF in cases of unilateral infarction is that damage in one hemisphere causes reduction of blood flow and metabolism in that area with consequent reduction of metabolism, and hence reduction of blood flow on the contralateral side. (p. 246)

Fujishima, Tanaka, Takeya, and Amae (1974) found bilateral reduction in blood flow in 13 of 29 patients and noted that for those patients with impaired consciousness during early stages post-onset of brain damage, the reduced blood flow persisted for more than two months.

Another dysfunction associated with acute lesions and which is intricately related to the reductions in blood flow is the release of neurotransmitters. In a study of 32 patients with subacute cerebral infarction, Meyer et al. (1970), found abnormal levels of neurotransmitter substances during the first two to three weeks post-onset which thereafter declined as the patient demonstrated clinical improvement. Moreover, patients with more severe neurological lesions tended to have higher levels of these substances. The patients also were found to have abnormal reduction of blood flow in both infarcted and noninfarcted hemispheres, suggesting that the substances contributed to the adverse pathophysiological effects, including reductions of blood flow, progression of cerebral infarction, and disordered cerebral metabolism.

The restitution of function is tied to the reestablishment of blood flow and reduction of neurotransmitters. This is summed up by Rubens (1977):

> It is clear that the disappearance of cerebral edema, bilateral reduction of cerebral blood flow, and abnormal concentrations of various transmitters

and other pharmocologically active substances yet to be identified play an
important role in spontaneous recovery. (p. 32)

Blood flow and metabolic dysfunction associated with acute lesions are
importantly related to the production of *diaschisis*. Diaschisis was proposed
by von Monakaw (1914) as a decreased functioning of intact neurons due
to the loss of neurophysiological influences from damaged or lost neurons
functionally tied to the intact neurons by neuroanatomical pathways. He
proposed that physiological recovery of the patient was due to the diminish-
ing effects of diachisis. Meyer et al. (1970, 1974) suggested that diaschisis
may be due to bilateral reductions in blood flow and release of neurotransmitters into brain tissue. Consequently the reduction of these cerebral disturbances brings about diminished effects of diaschisis and improved
functioning of the patient. The importance of diaschisis to recovery was
noted by Rubens (1977):

> Whatever its pathophysiology, diaschisis is an important phenomenon, one
> which is probably responsible for the greater part of what we call spontane-
> ous recovery in the first several months post-onset. (p. 32)

The time course of neural physiological changes following occlusive cerebrovascular accident (CVA) and the relationship of the changes to recovery
of communicative function are shown in Figure 3–1. Variations in these
changes would be expected as a function of the type and extent of lesion.

Although the ameliorative effects of physiological recovery associated
with the reduction of diaschisis serve as a primary mechanism for improved
function, other physiological and reorganizational changes have been
proposed to account for recovery. Luria (1963) hypothesized three explanations for return of function following brain damage: (1) shift of function to
homologous areas of the nondominant hemisphere, (2) recovery of injured
tissues, and (3) a reorganization of neural function permitting different
neuronal structures to assume the impaired functions. Each of these explanations will be examined, but it must be remembered that incontrovertible
evidence is not available to support any of the three and that all of the
mechanisms may be responsible for restitution.

Nondominant Hemisphere Participation in Recovery There is
some agreement that the right (nondominant) hemisphere has linguistic
capabilities and may be responsible for some posttrauma language recovery.
Questions remain, however, as to how much and under what circumstances
it is involved. Naeser, Hayward, Laughlin, Becker, Jernigan, and Zatz (1981)
demonstrated that although it is not as dramatic, the nondominant hemisphere also suffers a physiological (or morphological) reaction to a localized
lesion in the dominant hemisphere. The effects of such *bilateral* changes may
contribute to both the inability to predict disorder characteristics from

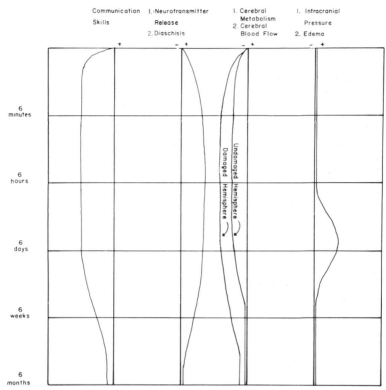

| Communication
Skills | 1. Neurotransmitter
Release
2. Diaschisis | 1. Cerebral
Metabolism
2. Cerebral
Blood Flow | 1. Intracranial
Pressure
2. Edema |

FIGURE 3–1 Hypothetical schematic diagram of relationship between neural physiological changes and recovery of communicative functioning. Reorganizational changes are not included because their time course is unknown. Variations would be expected as a function of type and extent of lesion. Diagram reflects typical occlusive CVA.

knowledge of lesion site and size (Naeser, Hayward, Laughlin, and Zatz, 1981), but also to uncertainty concerning the right hemisphere's participation in language recovery. Goldstein (1948) has pointed out the ubiquitous role of the right hemisphere in recovery of language: "... the minor cerebral hemisphere assumes the function of the major in language with great facility in some instances, with difficulty in others, and not at all in some persons" (p. 53). The evidence for right hemisphere participation in recovery derives from several sources. The purpose here is to provide a brief review of the types of evidence available, rather than to review the large body of data on functional hemispheric asymmetries.

First, supportive data is available from intracarotid injection of amobarbital in aphasic patients. Kinsbourne (1971) found that injection into the left carotid artery did not bring about an arrest of speech in three aphasic patients. When the right carotid artery was injected in two of these patients, all speech, including vocalization, was arrested; however comprehension was not affected. Kinsbourne (1975) proposed that the nondominant hemi-

73

sphere develops linguistic decoding skills in the emerging specialization of hemispheric function. These skills spring into action when the inhibitory effects of the dominant hemisphere, which attempts to jealously guard its linguistic preeminence, are inactivated by left brain damage. In terms of encoding Kinsbourne suggested that the nondominant hemisphere is not an active participant in normal speaking and, therefore, time is required to build up speech output programs in the minor hemisphere or to displace competing dominant hemisphere neural connections at the brainstem. Furthermore he hypothesized that the damaged dominant hemisphere may continue a minimal functional linguistic activity at a level below that of the minor hemisphere while at the same time inhibiting participation of the minor hemisphere in linguistic functions. This reasoning is supported by Moscovitch (1975, 1976) who noted that right hemisphere function is demonstrated only when the inhibitory effects of the dominant hemisphere are weakened or removed but that the left hemisphere damage is usually not sufficient to release these right hemisphere functions. He found that ". . . in most circumstances the aphasic performance reflects only the competence of the left hemisphere. The right hemisphere, being under the control of the left, can contribute little under these circumstances" (p. 595).

Dichotic listening studies provide a second source of evidence. Johnson, Sommers, and Weidner (1977) found a statistically significant left ear advantage in aphasic patients with left hemisphere brain damage. They also noted that there was a direct relationship between aphasic severity amd magnitude of left ear advantage; the greater the aphasic impairment, the larger the left ear advantage. Similarly Pettit and Noll (1979) found a significant left ear preference for 25 aphasic adults on digits and animal name dichotic tasks. In retesting at two months, they found that the left ear and aphasia test error scores had decreased. They concluded that ". . . the right hemisphere becomes the dominant hemisphere for speech when damage to the left hemisphere occurs. Further, the results tend to support the hypothesis that the right hemisphere improves in performance as language recovery takes place" (p. 198).

A third source of data is available from clinical reports. Nielsen (1946), for example, reported the case of a 66-year-old woman who suffered left cerebral hemisphere trauma with aphasia and who was again rendered aphasic by a right cerebrovascular accident nine years later. He concluded that ". . . there can be no doubt that her speech for the nine years was carried on by the right motor speech area. The case is therefore crucial as proving in this case the capacity of the minor motor speech areas to take over the function when the corresponding area on the left side was destroyed" (p. 150). Right hemisphere assumption of language recovery also has been documented in complete destruction of the language representation areas of the left hemisphere. Cummings, Benson, Walsh, and Levine (1979) presented a case study in which an embolic infarction destroyed the classical speech and language zones in a 54-year-old, right-handed man. The patient was severely aphasic. When reevaluated two and a half years later, his communicative abilities were significantly improved, particularly in comprehension but also in naming. Since the left hemisphere language representation areas were destroyed, Cummings et al. concluded that the right hemisphere was responsible for the recovery. Similarly Geschwind (1974) reported the case of a man who suffered brain damage and aphasia with recovery 18 years before his death. Postmortem examination of his brain revealed total destruction of the left perisylvian regions—the entire classical speech areas. Consequently the primary recovery would be attributed to right hemisphere assumption of a linguistic function.

A final source of data is the reports of patients who have undergone left hemispherectomies due to cerebral gliomas (Gott, 1973; Smith, 1979) or commissurotomies (Gazzaniga and Hillyard, 1971; Gazzaniga and Sperry, 1967). The immediate effect of a left hemispherectomy is to render the patient severely aphasic with auditory comprehension limited to perhaps only the ability to follow simple commands. Performance in comprehension appears to improve with time, but production is severely limited. Commissurotomized patients have been used to investigate capacities and functions of the right hemisphere. In general these split brain subjects never appear to develop language in the right hemisphere beyond the ability to carry out simple commands and to recognize objects and assign names to them. These nonexpressive functions and some small amount of automatic speech, such as cursing and counting, are all that can confidently be attributed to the right hemisphere. The language abilities of the right hemisphere, then, appear limited in these patients and are summed up by Moscovitch (1976): "Removal of the left hemisphere control either by commissurotomy or hemispherectomy leads to a level of right hemisphere linguistic performance that exceeds that of normal people and of about half the aphasics with healthy right hemispheres" (p. 97). This performance appears limited, however, and is perhaps best summarized by Collins (1976) who reviewed the literature and observed that no significant speech and language functioning has followed dominant hemispherectomy.

In summary, the theoretical framework for right hemisphere assumption of language recovery is as follows: The right hemisphere develops language capabilities along with the dominant but is gradually inhibited by the left hemisphere as these skills are progressively displaced to and controlled by the left. Dominant hemisphere brain damage, if sufficient in magnitude, releases the previously inhibited linguistic capacities of the right hemisphere. The recovery attributable to the right hemisphere is seldom equivalent to its linguistic capabilities because the left hemisphere, even when severely damaged, continues to jealously guard its linguistic prerogatives and inhibit the right. The magnitude of the recovery due to right hemisphere activity is perhaps limited to the language abilities of hemispherectomy patients and is therefore not great, despite the clinical reports of significant language recovery in severe left hemisphere brain damage.

Left Hemisphere Bases of Recovery As noted earlier, two additional physiological bases of recovery are a restitution of injured tissues and a reorganization of neural function permitting different neuronal structures to assume the impaired functions. Data relative to recovery of tissue damage has already been noted: Abnormal levels of neurotransmitter substances are reduced, cerebral blood flow is reestablished, collateral circulation is developed, and diachisis lessens which would be expected to be related to early stages of the recovery process. Coupled to these physiological processes are changes at the cellular level which have been demonstrated in the central nervous system of mammals undergoing induced lesions. Moore (1974) reviewed data relative to axonal collateral sprouting and reinnervation in animals and noted:

> It is certainly a component of the central nervous system's response to injury and one which may well participate in the phenomena of recovery of function. The dogma that regeneration does not occur in the mammalian central nervous system and contribute to recovery of function should be put aside in favor of further experimentation. (pp. 123–124)

He noted further, however, that

> . . . there is no instance known in which restitution of anatomic integrity occurs after destruction of central axons within the mammalian central nervous system. For this reason, regenerative sprouting cannot be used as a basis for recovery of function after central lesions although it may participate to some extent as a component of recovery phenomena. (p. 123)

The recovery of injured tissue would be expected to be an early stage in the recovery process. Tied up with it and continuing for longer periods of time post-onset of brain damage are reorganizational changes that relate to the assumption of lost functions by different neuronal structures.

Evidence which suggests left hemisphere reorganizational changes derives from some of the same data bases as those which have yielded support for right hemisphere recovery processes: left hemisphere damage may generate a severe aphasia with recovery that does not equal the linguistic capacities of the right hemisphere. Conversely severe left hemisphere damage may yield improved function far beyond what might logically be expected to be within the capabilities of the right hemisphere. Stronger support comes from serial lesions in animals and man. Butters, Rosen, and Stein (1974) observed in serial lesions in monkeys that ". . . the present evidence implicates the cortex immediately adjacent to a serially ablated focus as well as more distant anterior and posterior association areas as mediators of recovery" (p. 462). For example, Geschwind (1974) described a human patient undergoing a series of surgical procedures for removal of a left hemisphere tumor. After each surgery the patient was rendered aphasic and then recovered only to become aphasic again with the next brain tissue removal.

In summary, the recovery process is complex, probably involves both left and right hemispheres, and operates on a continuum from earlier, more physiologically based changes to later neural reorganizational processes, although the exact time course is unclear. The weight of each of the hypothesized recovery mechanisms cannot be assigned because they are subject to individual variations related to the extent of cerebral lateralization; the etiology, extent, and site of lesion; and multiple hypothesized, but not yet documented, variables. What is known is that spontaneous recovery accounts for significant improvement in linguistic facility in the patient who has not received communicative rehabilitation.

spontaneous recovery

Spontaneous recovery is defined as return of function not attributable to therapeutic intervention and addresses the issue of improved speech and language facility due to physiological and reorganization changes. Several studies have explored the nature and extent of this recovery. Vignolo (1964) examined a group of 27 untreated aphasics. They were evaluated and then reevaluated with a minimum of 40 days between the first and second testing. The time of initial testing varied from less than one month to more than six months post-onset of brain damage. Of the 27 patients, 15 changed between first and second testing, 14 improved, and one deteriorated. Twelve of the patients did not change. When the time post-onset was considered, it was found that a higher percentage of patients with improved function had been first evaluated within two months of brain damage and that the percentage of improved patients decreased with the time interval from brain damage to first testing. Vignolo also noted that ". . . the end of the second month represents a turning point in the course of the disturbance. Indeed, it appears as if any degree of spontaneous restitution could occur in subjects examined for the first time within two months from onset, no matter how severely affected they are" (pp. 379–380).

Culton (1969) examined two groups of patients for eight weeks. Group I was composed of 19 patients who had incurred brain damage less than 30 days before testing. Group II included patients who had been aphasic for from 11 to 48 months and who had undergone language rehabilitation. A test battery, composed of reading, writing, auditory comprehension and oral expression tasks, and a measure of nonverbal intelligence, was administered at two-week intervals. Results revealed that the Group II patients were highly stable in their test performance during the entire test period, while Group I patients demonstrated improved functioning on all tasks, with one exception, at each test interval. Improved performance was most evident between the first and second test administrations. Culton observed:

> Rapid spontaneous recovery of language function was noted in the first month following the onset of aphasia. Although an increase in mean scores was noted, further significant improvement was not evident during the second month. This is somewhat incompatible with the predominant notion that significant spontaneous recovery of language function continues to occur three to six months after the onset of aphasia. (p. 831)

Sarno and Levita (1971) first administered the Functional Communication Profile to a group of 28 right-handed, right hemiplegic, and aphasic patients within two days of brain damage; they then tested 18 of the patients at three months and tested 14 of the patients again at six months. The attrition in the sample was primarily due to mortality. Comparison of profile values revealed greater improvement during the zero- to three-month period than during the three- to six-month interval. Findings from these three studies cannot be directly compared regardless of the measurement device used because of differences in test interval time. The findings are consistent, however, with the findings of spontaneous improvement in communication skills in ten males as measured by the Minnesota Test for the Differential Diagnosis of Aphasia by Hagen (1973). This study revealed that there was improved performance for the untreated patients for the first three months post-onset of brain damage but not thereafter without treatment. The results are also consistent with the findings of Lomas and Kertesz (1978) who investigated 31 untreated patients within thirty days of onset and at three months using the Western Aphasia Battery. Even when divided into four groups based on perturbations of high and low fluency and comprehension, all four groups improved significantly during the three-month period.

A final empirical data base for spontaneous recovery is a follow-up study of the earlier Vignolo investigation by Basso, Capitani, and Vignolo (1979) utilizing comparable procedures. Results confirmed the earlier findings— that is, patients first evaluated at less than two months post onset of brain damage included a larger percentage who improved than did groups first tested at between two and six months or more than six months.

Perhaps the only major statement that might be made about these six groups of empirical data is that a decelerating curve of improvement appears to be coincident with spontaneous physiological restorative and reorganizational processes subsequent to brain damage. The slope of the curve would be expected to be dictated by the status of the brain. If one major lacuna were to be identified, it would be the almost complete absence of information on this relationship between physiological and communicative aspects of recovery. Almost no research appears to be directed toward, for example, language recovery and cerebral blood flow or language recovery and abnormal levels of neurotransmitter substances following central nervous system lesions. However, there are two exceptions. Kohlmeyer (1976) studied the relationship between the site of vascular lesion, type of aphasia, and spontaneous recovery investigated by clinico-neuropsychological and neuroradiological methods. He found that the first 10 to 14 days seemed decisive. Severe persisting deficits after this time were indicative of a very poor prognosis for recovery. Unfortunately the composition of the language test battery was not reported, and it is difficult to evaluate specifically the reported complete recovery in one-third of all Broca's aphasics within two weeks subsequent to occlusion of the internal carotid artery, since no test results were reported.

Jabbari, Maulsby, Holtzapple, and Marshall (1979) examined the relationship between EEG and Porch Index of Communicative Ability (PICA) scores in 44 right-handed male patients. Neurological testing and PICA administration were completed first at two to four weeks post-onset of stroke and then at four- to six-month intervals. EEG was performed within two weeks of onset and repeated with the PICA and neurological examinations. It was found that EEG and PICA curves were highly related. This relationship was most notable in patients with the largest amount of language improvement. Little EEG improvement was noted in patients with moderate to severe aphasia.

The length of spontaneous recovery is not known. Estimates have varied from one month to years. To a large extent, the accuracy of determining the time frame is dictated by the measures that serve as inferential estimators of change and the definition of what constitutes "significant" improvement. It is perhaps safe to say that, in the majority of patients who have become aphasic secondary to cerebrovascular accident, the primary spontaneous recovery occurs within one month, although additional, more limited improvement may be seen up to one year or more post-onset.

Determining accurately the extent and limits of spontaneous recovery is critical for two reasons. First, because it may be indicative of the total recovery with or without treatment. Sarno and Levita (1971) observed:

> Spontaneous recovery has sometimes been equated with physiologic stabilization and it may well be that the physiologic factors associated with the natural recovery process may define the potential limits within which residual function can actually be achieved. (p. 175)

Spontaneous recovery is also important for determining the efficiency of speech and language rehabilitation. It must serve as the reference against which all treatment is compared because it is indicative of improvement not attributable to clinical efforts. If physiological recovery can be predicted and factored from total improvement scores with significant residual recovery remaining assignable to treatment, the value of treatment will be demonstrated.

If physiological variables determine the limits of residual function, speech-language pathologists will not be fortunate for their role will need to be redefined in the clinical setting. If improvement significantly exceeds physiological recovery, they will be fortunate because many years of intensive work with brain-damaged patients will not be ruled as of limited value with all the implications that a finding of this type engenders. The effects of therapy have been studied and directly address the issue of the efficacy of treatment.

○ THE EFFICACY OF TREATMENT

There is some question as to whether the therapy procedures for the aphasic patient are of value or if the patient gets better as a result of treatment or in spite of it. Not all patients are candidates for individualized treatment, and part of the problem of establishing the value of the invested time and effort is that no completely reliable methods are available for determining which patients will benefit from which treatments. There is little question that patients improve with treatment, but as observed by Sarno (1976), "The questions which must be asked are: how much, in what way, under what circumstances, and to what end" (p. 256). Darley (1972), in a review of treatment efficacy, succinctly described the questions that need to be answered:

> 1.   Does language rehabilitation accomplish measurable gains in language function beyond what can be expected to occur as a result of spontaneous recovery? Or, stated differently, does therapy have a decisive influence on the course of recovery and the ultimate outcome?
>
> 2.   Are the language gains attributable to therapy worth the necessary investment of time, effort and money?
>
> 3.   What are the relative degrees of effectiveness of various modes of treatment of aphasia? (pp. 4–5)

Darley reviewed the accumulated research on the effectiveness of treatment and concluded:

> The data are not consistent, but the populations sampled have been different in many respects. One is led to the conclusion that any all-inclusive statement about the efficacy of aphasia would be ill-advised. Apparently, many statements are necessary—that is, separate statements about different kinds of aphasic patients, and different with regard to several dimensions (pp. 7–8).

Darley also noted that there perhaps would never be one complete definitive study. Similarly Holland (1975) observed that no single study could ever establish the efficacy of treatment. These conclusions of Holland and Darley appear to suggest a research plan reminiscent of the methodology needed to establish the construct validity of a test. The construct validity of a test can never be completely established, but the weight of accumulated evidence aids in determining its utility for a particular purpose.

In Darley's (1972) review of efficacy, he detailed the criteria for further studies:

> ... the proposed investigations of the efficacy of language therapy must include specification of the nature of the language disorders treated; selection of a suitable control group; scrutiny of clearly specified periods during the initial recovery phase or following it; provision of objective measurement of relevant aspects of the behavior change; and specification of the nature, intensity, duration, and quality of the therapy. (p. 14.)

He also noted that the following subject selection parameters be considered: (1) age of patient at the onset of aphasia; (2) educational level, social status, and prior language status; (3) intelligence; (4) health during recovery; (5) social milieu of the patient; (6) etiology of aphasia; (7) site and extent of lesion; (8) time between onset of aphasia and institution of therapy; (9) the type of aphasia; and (10) nonlanguage behavioral characteristics.

Unfortunately the efficacy studies completed since Darley's 1972 review have not met his hope that

> ... researchers can introduce a richness of description and a rigor or procedure which they might be careless about otherwise ... (and so by doing) ... increase the likelihood that 10 years hence the profession will enjoy substantial agreement about the nature of language breakdown and what can best be done about it. (pp. 19–20)

Several recent studies will be examined to update knowledge regarding the efficacy of treatment.

The first group of data is from Smith (1972). Subjects were evaluated on subtests of the Minnesota Test for the Differential Diagnosis of Aphasia and audiological and neuropsychological batteries. Patient clinical data was quantified in great detail including age, presence of associated motor and sensory deficits, type of lesion, education, handedness, and occupation. Four groups were identified:

Group I: 67 poststroke patients with aphasia of at least three months' duration on which test-retest comparisons were used to determine the initial effects of therapy.

Group II: 24 of the 67 poststroke patients of Group I examined a third time an average of 20.6 months postdischarge from treatment.

Group III: 15 patients examined at the initiation of therapy and at a follow-up period who did not undergo intensive speech therapy.

Group IV: 13 patients with aphasia due to trauma who had received intensive therapy.

Treatment was described as follows:

> Each received a minimum of five hours of individual and group therapy
> daily for at least five weeks (125 hours). The therapists were graduate
> students, most with no prior experience in aphasia therapy.
>
> They were supervised by clinicians with experience varying from one to
> four years. Individual programs of therapy were designed by the students
> and clinicians and administered to each aphasic by three or four students.
> Although the supervising clinician for each aphasic was usually constant,
> the student therapists usually changed after each five (summer) or ten (fall
> and winter) week terms. (Smith, 1972, pp. 99–100)

Given the care with which this study was carried out, it is surprising that
this statement includes the entire description of the therapy provided. Nevertheless the treatment effects were significant since the untreated group
demonstrated only negligible changes in language test scores whereas the
67 stroke patients and 13 traumatic aphasics showed marked improvement
in all language functions after the period of intensive therapy. If it is remembered that most of the spontaneous physiological recovery would have taken
place before therapy was begun, these results are impressive. It should be
pointed out, however, that the control and experimental groups were not
equivalent. The untreated patients were older, less well educated, more
severely impaired in language and nonlanguage functions, and included a
higher proportion of patients with bilateral involvement.

Perhaps the best-controlled study of treatment value is the Veterans
Administration investigation undertaken in 1973 (Wertz, Brookshire, Holtzapple, Hubbard, Porch, and West, 1974) and reported five years later in
preliminary form (Wertz, Collins, Weiss, Brookshire, Friden, Kurtzke, and
Pierce, 1978). Since the study appears to be the most carefully undertaken
a priori study of its kind, it bears specific scrutiny. Subjects were selected
according to the following criteria: sustained a single left hemisphere
thromboembolic cerebrovascular accident, entered the study at four weeks
post-onset of brain damage, aged between 40 and 80 years, scored between
the fifteenth and seventy-fifth percentile on the Porch Index of Communicative Ability, had premorbid ability to read English and no major sensory
(auditory, visual, tactile) deficits or related medical problems. More than
1,000 patients were screened, but only 67 met all criteria and were entered
into the study. With a subject selection attrition of this magnitude, it is
questionable whether the sample was representative of the aphasic population in most clinical facilities. Nevertheless since the purposes of the study
were to document the amount and rate of language improvement associated
with two different types of treatment and not necessarily to determine the
efficacy of treatment, the results are important.

Patients were randomly assigned to one of two groups: Group A, which
was provided with "traditional" speech and language therapy for 44 weeks,

or Group B, which received "nontraditional" treatment emphasizing problem solving but not involving manipulation of speech and language variables for 44 weeks. Patients in Group A received four hours of individual clinician-directed therapy and four hours of machine-assisted therapy each week, and patients of Group B participated in four hours of group therapy and four hours of recreational therapy a week. The same therapists provided treatment for each group. Some detail regarding the content of the therapy was described (Wertz et al., 1974), but since it was necessary for treatment to be tailored to the patient's communicative impairment, at least for Group A, the treatments are best characterized as principles rather than specific methods.

At 4, 15, 26, 37, and 48 weeks post-onset of brain damage, each patient was evaluated on a battery of measures, including a neurological examination, sensory screening, the PICA, Token Test, a word fluency measure, a motor speech evaluation, a test of nonverbal intelligence, a rating of functional language use, and a rating of conversational ability. However only approximately 50 percent of the subjects completed the 44 weeks of treatment with primary attrition due to factors such as distance between home and the treatment center. To maintain the data base, the initial sample was separated into four cohorts, defined by the number of weeks of treatment received. Therefore patients who had been seen for the full 48 weeks also were represented in the cohorts at 15, 26, and 37 weeks. Patients who dropped out earlier were included in less treatment cohorts.

Results were reported primarily for the PICA, although both groups at each measurement point made significant gains on most of the other measures. Communicative ability as measured by the PICA improved significantly for each group at each measurement time during the treatment period. Most of the overall improvement occurred during the first 11 weeks of treatment, but gains were still observable during later therapy intervals. Group A (individually treated) patients showed a gradual decline in the amount of improvement for succeeding treatment segments, whereas Group B subjects showed greater improvement during the third treatment period (26 to 37 weeks) than during the second (15 to 26 weeks). Differences in improvement between groups were few, limited to differences in PICA scores, and generally in favor of the individually treated patients. Improvement continued beyond the 26-week measurement point, suggesting that recovery was probably due to the treatment for the later stages of the study since spontaneous recovery would be expected to have run its course.

This study has important implications. The expected improvement as a function of time and treatment is not surprising since the study by Sarno, Silverman, and Sands (1970) is the only major a priori investigation that has not found differences. Despite the subject attrition problem, the most important findings of this study were left mostly unstated—that is, the group-treated patients' recovery was not significantly different from the individually treated subjects except in terms of PICA scores. The most important findings were that the two groups *did not* differ significantly in their performance on the Token Test, a word fluency measure, a motor speech evaluation, the Coloured Progressive Matrices, a conversation ability measure, or an informant's rating of functional language use. Moreover, it is noteworthy that at the last two measurement points of the study (37 and 48 weeks), there were small differences in the intake PICA percentiles for the two groups (three and six percentile points, respectively) that could account for at least a part of the greater improvement for the individually treated patients.

The small differences in improvement between the two groups did not go unnoticed, however. Wertz et al. (1978) observed:

> Our results indicate that individual treatment may be slightly superior to group treatment; however, the cost effective advantage of group therapy should prompt speech pathologists to consider it for, at least, a part of a patient's care. (p. 15)

A third study was completed by Sarno and Levita (1979) who investigated the effect of time on the recovery course of treated aphasic patients. Subjects were 34 patients with first episode left hemisphere vascular lesions selected from a pool of 1,730 consecutive admissions to a major medical center. All were right-handed native speakers of English. They were assigned to one of three groups—fluent, nonfluent, or global—based upon clinical testing that included the Boston Diagnostic Aphasia Examination. A test battery composed of the Functional Communication Profile and subtests of the Neurosensory Center Comprehensive Examination of Aphasia (token, visual naming, sentence repetition, and word fluency tests) was administered at 4, 8, 12, 26 and 52 weeks poststroke with an allowable variation of plus or minus one week. Patients received three to five sessions of therapy per week based on a "stimulation-pedagogical approach," although the amount of therapy decreased as the time poststroke increased. Comparison on the measures completed at 4 and 52 weeks revealed significant improvement only on the Functional Communication Profile, although the general trend was improvement on each of the tests used. When considered from onset, the extent of recovery became less as time progressed. Interestingly the fluent aphasics demonstrated the greatest gains and the global aphasics the least during the first six months, whereas during the last half of the year the global aphasics demonstrated the greatest gains and the fluent aphasics the least as measured by the Functional Communication Profile. The nonfluent aphasics demonstrated the least amount of improvement of the three groups from 3 to 12 months, the treatment period in which spontaneous recovery would not be expected to have a significant effect on test scores.

The three studies reviewed appear to be the major a priori investigations completed since Darley's review. Several other investigators, however, have taken retrospective (*post hoc*) looks at treatment effects.

Kertesz and McCabe (1977) were interested in patterns of spontaneous recovery and in prognosis rather than the impact of treatment, but they made comparisons between treated and untreated patients. Ninety-three subjects, divided into four overlapping groups, were evaluated by means of the Western Aphasia Battery (Kertesz and Poole, 1974) within six weeks of onset of brain damage and at three months, six months, and then at yearly intervals. Virtually no information on the type of treatment was provided. Results revealed that, in general, the greatest improvement occurred between onset and three months, although additional gains were evident during subsequent intervals. Moreover no significant differences were observed between untreated and treated global and Broca's aphasics, although the samples of these patients were very small at each measurement interval. For example, no more than five patients were within these classifications at any of the measurement points, and in fact, no treated Broca's aphasics were evaluated within 45 days of onset of brain damage. The lack of a detailed specification of therapy and the small samples do not allow any conclusions regarding the effectiveness of treatment.

Deal and Deal (1978) investigated five groups of post–cerebrovascular accident aphasic patients in a retrospective review of treatment effectiveness. Subjects were evaluated and treatment initiated during the first month (Group I—17 patients), second month (Group II—9 patients), third month (Group III—9 patients), or fourth through seventh months (Group IV—10 patients) post-onset. Patients in Group V were evaluated the first month post-onset but were not treated due to the unavailability of services. The patients in each of the treatment groups received at least 24 therapy visits over at least a two-month interval. Initial and 12-month Porch Index of Communicative Ability scores were obtained for all but 13 patients. Multiple t-tests were used to compare the initial scores and 12-month scores between groups and the differences between initial and 12-month scores within each group. Scores were not significantly different at initial testing, but at 12 months performance was better for the Group I compared to the Group V patients but for none of the other group comparisons. Within-group comparisons were all significant. Moreover the patients who were treated early (first three months post-onset of brain damage) changed more than the untreated patients or those for whom treatment was initiated late (fourth through seventh month post-onset).

Similar findings were reported by Basso et al. (1979). They investigated the effects of treatment in 281 aphasic patients (162 treated, 119 untreated) who were evaluated in terms of oral expression, auditory comprehension, reading, and writing and were then rated on the basis of this testing on a zero to four severity scale for each modality. Subjects were divided on the parameters of time between onset and initial testing (two months or less, two to six months, more than six months), type of aphasia (fluent, disfluent), aphasia severity (moderate, severe), and rehabilitation (treated, untreated). At a point at least six months after the first examination, the patients were retested on the same measures. For treated patients, only those were included who received no less than three individual therapy sessions a month for at least five consecutive months. Therapy consisted of 45- to 50-minute sessions of a "stimulation" type supplemented by homework and group meetings. The untreated patients did not receive services because of family or transportation problems. *Improvement* was defined as an increase of at least two points on the severity scale between the first and second examinations. Patients who did not progress or improved only one point on the scale were termed *unchanged.*

Statistical analyses revealed significant differences for time, severity, and rehabilitation—that is, treated patients demonstrated greater improvement than did untreated patients; patients treated early progressed more than those treated late post-onset; and moderately involved treated patients exhibited greater gains than did severe patients. No differences were found between fluent and nonfluent aphasics.

What might be concluded from the investigations of treatment efficacy? First, it appears that the restitution of function associated with treatment follows a time course similar to that of spontaneous recovery—the most pronounced improvement occurs immediately post-onset and then decreases in magnitude, in most cases, with time. However since randomly selected patients have not been assigned to nontreatment groups in investigations to date, it is not possible to determine progress attributable to treatment or, stated conversely, to factor out the effects of physiological recovery.

Second, the effects of treatment appear to be quantitative rather than qualitative. Improved performance is associated with intensive treatment, but treated patients do not appear to have, for example, differential improvement in reading or auditory comprehension compared to untreated patients. However the data in this area is meager, and some studies (Sarno and Levita, 1979; Wertz et al., 1978) suggest that improvement may be observable on some measures but not others. Furthermore it is not possible to determine if these findings are a function of the differences in patient performance or the assessment validity of the measures used.

Third, no definitive statements can be made regarding the value of different treatment approaches. The almost complete absence of description of the therapy content is striking and none of the studies is replicable, except, perhaps, for that of Wertz et al. (1978). Therefore, treatment appears to generate greater gains than no treatment, but the type of therapy, if competently performed to address important aspects of the patient's communicative impairment, has not yet been demonstrated to be a critical factor in recovery. This is not to say that some types of therapy do not produce significantly greater gains than other types but, rather, to point out that these differences have not yet been shown from group studies.

In terms of treatment efficacy, then, some progress has been made in providing a data base to serve as scaffolding for verifying the importance of treatment (a summary of efficacy studies is presented in Table 3–1). However, the criteria specified by Darley as prerequisites for a definitive study have not been met, and his questions, "Can significant gains attributable to treatment be demonstrated?" and "What are the relative degrees of effectiveness of different modes of treatment?," remain only partially answered. His third question, "Are treatment effects worth the time, effort, and money?," is tied up with the clinical enterprise of prognosis, the next topic of discussion.

○ PROGNOSIS

Recovery studies supply important information regarding identification of factors that are predictive of the patient's final level of performance. These factors, or prognostic indicators, can aid in making decisions about who to treat and how to construct the therapy regime. Each of the factors will be reviewed here with the purpose of establishing and evaluating the rationale for their inclusion as predictors.

Prognostic indicators are implicitly viewed as independent or dependent, linear or dichotomous, and accumulative and/or interactive. Examples may serve to clarify these concepts. Motivation might be considered a relatively *independent* variable. It does not appear to be affected by age, cerebral dominance, amount of brain damage, severity of aphasia, or education, and it evolves from the emotional and psychological resources of the individual which are difficult to predict or measure. Severity of aphasia, on the other hand, is *dependent* on the site and extent of brain damage. Age, as it is customarily measured in years, is *linear* although the physiological changes associated with it are not, as will be discussed later. Factors such as etiology are frequently *dichotomous*—the origin of the brain damage, for example, is traumatic, cerebrovascular, or neoplastic. Prognostic variables, if considered *accumulative,* can be added. Therefore, a severe aphasia in an elderly patient would generate a lower level of predicted recovery than would a young patient with severe aphasia or an older patient with a mild aphasia. *Interactions* between variables are also to be expected. For example, the effects of age and extent of lesion may be greater than the predicted cumulative weight of the two parameters considered individually.

One framework for classifying prognostic indicators is in terms of prominence—that is, as primary, secondary or tertiary factors (see Table 3–2). *Primary* indicators include site, etiology, and extent of brain damage; age; cerebral dominance; cerebrovascular circulation; time since onset of brain damage; and any other factors that relate specifically to neural function. *Secondary* indicators are end products of the brain damage. Included are type and severity of communicative impairment and presence or absence of

TABLE 3-1

Summary of Recent Data-Based Studies of Treatment Efficacy

STUDY	SUBJECTS	TESTS	MEASUREMENT (periods)	TREATMENT	RESULTS
Butfield and Zangwill (1946)	66 acquired aphasic subjects. *Group 1* (52 patients): Treatment initiated less than six months post-onset of brain damage. *Group 2* (14 patients): Treatment initiated after six months post-onset.	Speech, reading, writing, and calculation rated as mild, moderate, or severe.	Severity at initation of treatment; degree of improvement (much improved, improved, unchanged) at termination of treatment.	Individually constructed reeducational programs. Two ½ hour sessions per week. Total sessions varied from 5 to 290.	Speech "Much improved" in 40% of severe, 56% of moderate and 58% of mild patients. Speech "unchanged" in 34%. Less marked improvement for reading, writing, and calculation.
Wepman (1951)	68 aphasic patients at least six months post-onset of traumatic brain damage. Mean age 25.8 years.	Wechsler-Bellevue Test of Adult Intelligence, Progressive Achievement Test, Halstead Aphasia Screening test.	Intelligence and achievement testing at referral and at conclusion of treatment.	Educational training in reading, writing, spelling, and mathematics; speech therapy based on stimulation approach. Treatment program included classes which met 6 hours per day, 5 days a week, for 18 months.	Educational level (from achievement test results) increased by 5.3 years. Speech improved by two levels on a five-point scale which ranged from no speech to normal or average expression. When progress was categorized, 51 percent were "much improved," 35 percent were "improved," and 14 percent were "unchanged."
Marks, Taylor, and Rusk (1957)	324 patients ranging in age from less than 20 to more than 60 years old (63% more than 50 years old).	Psychological evaluation, Halstead-Wepman aphasia screening test, patient and family interviews, and evaluation of functional language skills at initiation of	Test battery at entry to study. Rating scale of improvement (excellent, good, fair, poor) at end of rehabilitation at facility. Evaluation of progress made by three	Number of therapy sessions varied from none to 110. Twenty percent had no therapy; 39.5% had more than 21. Sessions were 30 minutes in length. Pragmatic	Of the patients treated, 6.9% made excellent progress, 32% good, 21.4% fair, and 49.7% poor.

Vignolo (1964)	69 aphasic adults. 42 who received treatment; 27 who did not. Non-treated patients older and less educated.	study. Rating of improvement at completion of rehabilitation. Oral description, oral naming, and comprehension of commands rated as good, sufficient for communication, poor, or nil.	speech-language pathologists. Minimum interval of 40 days between initial testing and posttesting.	stimulation-based treatment employed. Sixty-eight percent of patients not treated or treated for two or less months. Minimum of 20 therapy sessions in not less than 40 days with at least one session per week. Therapy was primarily by a stimulation approach.	Comparison of improvement between groups not significant. However trend toward greater improvement and frequency of recovery in treated group. Concluded that training extending over at least six months is effective.
Schuell, Jenkins, and Jimenez-Pabon (1964)	73 patients divided according to prognostic group.	Minnesota Test for Differential Diagnosis of Aphasia.	At initiation and termination of treatment. Time interval ranged from one to 13 months. Mean interval of 3 months.	Stimulation therapy. Length and number of sessions unspecified.	Significant reduction in error percentages in most of the five major sections of the Minnesota Test (9 of 10 tests of auditory comprehension; 7 of 11 tests of visual and reading disturbances; 16 of 20 speech and language tests; 14 of 14 writing tests; 7 of 8 numerical and arithmetic tests.
Beyn and Shokhor-Trotskaya (1966)	25 patients with "motor" aphasia resulting from cerebrovascular disease. Treatment initiated within one month of brain damage for 18 patients; between one and three months for 7 patients.	Not specified.	Not specified. Assumed to be at beginning and end of treatment.	"Preventive" therapy to limit development of telegraphic speech during recovery.	None of the patients developed a telegraphic style of oral expression. Sixteen demonstrated pronounced agrammatism in the agreement of the parts of the sentence and incompleteness of utterances, and 9 had difficulty in the use of prepositions at the final stages of treatment.

TABLE 3-1 (Continued)

STUDY	SUBJECTS	TESTS	MEASUREMENT (periods)	TREATMENT	RESULTS
Sands, Sarno, and Shankweiler (1969)	30 post-CVA aphasic patients. Median age 56.5 years.	Functional Communication Profile	Initial evaluation, re-evaluation at discharge and from 4 to 12 months posttreatment.	Daily therapy (type unspecified). Duration from 2 weeks to 2 years, 8 months (median = 7.5 months).	Median overall gain of 10% on FCP from initiation of treatment to discharge; 5% gain from discharge to post-treatment reevaluation.
Sarno, Silverman, and Sands (1970)	31 post-CVA patients with severe expressive-receptive aphasia (FCP < 31%) assigned to programmed instruction, nonprogrammed instruction, and no treatment groups. Mean age 64.8 years.	Functional Communication Profile. Ten tests designed to determine language residuals corresponding to the experimental tasks.	FCP administered at entry to study. Ten subtests administered before treatment, immediately after completion of teaching of specific terminal behavior, as a battery after completion of all terminal behaviors, and as a battery one month after completion of all treatments for treatment groups. As battery at entry to study and three months later for nontreatment group.	4 to 36 weeks of treatment (mean 17.1 weeks). Total treatment sessions ranged from 13 to 91 (mean 56 sessions or 28 hours) for treatment groups.	No significant difference between treatment groups on 8 of the 10 subsets on learning after therapy on each terminal behavior or on retention one month after completion of therapy. "There were no significant differences in outcome under the three treatment conditions."
Smith (1972)	Group 1: 67 aphasic adults three or more months post-onset of brain damage. Group 2: A subset of 24 subjects from Group 1. Group 3: 15 patients who did not receive treatment.	Comprehensive neuro-psychological battery including selected subtests of the Minnesota Test for the Differential Diagnosis of Aphasia and Wechsler Adult Intelligence Scale, among others.	Group 1 evaluated at initiation and termination of treatment. Group 2 evaluated additionally following discharge from therapy (Mean = 20.6 months). Group 3 evaluated at initiation of study and then retested a mean	Each treated patient received a minimum of five hours individual and group therapy a week for at least five weeks (125 hrs.).	Statistically significant gains for Group 1 patients on 27 of 28 language tests and 8 of 10 nonlanguage measures (however, percent gains were negligible on 6 measures). Similar findings for Group 4, but results were not statistically analyzed. Negligible

Reference	Subjects	Test	Timing	Treatment	Results
	Group 4: 13 patients with aphasia secondary to traumatic brain damage.		of 22.6 months later. *Group 4* tested at initiation and termination of treatment.		improvement in mean language scores of Group 3 patients (not treated).
Kertesz and McCabe (1977)	93 aphasic patients divided into four overlapping subgroups on the basis of initial and follow-up testing post-onset of brain damage.	Western Aphasia Battery	Initial testing within six weeks post-onset with retesting at three months, six months, and thereafter at year intervals.	Type and intensity of treatment unspecified.	"Although some cases recovered exceptionally well while under therapy, there was no significant difference between the treated and untreated groups, where such a comparison was possible."
Deal and Deal (1978)	*Group 1:* 17 patients evaluated and treatment initiated during the first month post-onset. *Group 2:* 9 patients evaluated and treatment initiated during second month post-onset. *Group 3:* 9 patients evaluated and treatment initiated during third month post-onset. *Group 4:* 10 patients evaluated and treatment initiated during fourth, fifth, sixth, or seventh month post-onset.	Porch Index of Communicative Ability	At initiation of therapy (for treated groups), one month post-onset (for untreated patients), and at termination or 12 months post-onset of brain damage.	At least 24 therapy visits over at least a two-month period. Type of therapy unspecified.	Significantly greater improvement in PICA scores for Group 1 than for Group 5. All other intergroup comparisons nonsignificant. Final PICA scores significantly higher than initial scores for all groups. However improvement was least for untreated patients. Change scores for Groups 1, 2, and 3 significantly different from those of Groups 4 and 5.
Wertz, Collins, Weiss, Brookshire, Friden, Kurtzke, and Pierce (1978)	67 aphasic subjects post–first episode left CVA between 40 and 80 years of age. PICA percentiles between 25 and 75. No	Neurological examination, sensory screening, PICA, Token Test, word fluency and motor speech measures, Raven Matrices, ratings of	4, 15, 26, 37, and 48 weeks post-onset of brain damage.	*Group A:* Four hours of clinician-directed and four hours of machine-assisted treatment per week. *Group B:* Four hours of	Significant improvement for each group at each measurement point on PICA. Significant gains on "...most other measures" as well at each test period.

TABLE 3-1 (Continued)

STUDY	SUBJECTS	TESTS	MEASUREMENT (periods)	TREATMENT	RESULTS
	major sensory deficits or related medical problems.	functional language use and conversational ability.		group therapy and four hours of recreational therapy a week.	Observable differences between groups only on the PICA in favor of individually treated patients.
Serno and Levita (1979)	34 patients with first episode CVA assigned to fluent, nonfluent, and global groups based on Boston Diagnostic Aphasia Examination.	Functional Communication Profile and subtests of the Neurosensory Center Comprehensive Examination of Aphasia.	4, 8, 12, 26, and 52 weeks post-onset of brain damage with allowable alteration of one week.	Three to five sessions per week based on "simulation-pedagogical" approach.	Comparison at 4 and 52 weeks showed significant improvement only on Functional Communication Profile. General trend of improvement on each of the measures used. Degree of improvement decreased with increase in time post-onset of brain damage.
Basso, Capitani, and Vignolo (1979)	281 aphasic patients (162 treated, 119 untreated). Mean age 50.2 years.	"Standard language examination" including tests of oral expression, auditory comprehension, writing, and reading. Tests interpreted as scaled ratings, 0–4, for each area tested.	Evaluated at referral and more than six months later unless language recovery completed earlier. Improvement defined as at least an increase of two points on scaled rating on second examination.	Treated group received at least three sessions of stimulation therapy per week for at least five months.	Significant improvement for treated patients for oral expression, auditory comprehension, reading, and writing.

TABLE 3-2

Prognostic Indicators for Neurogenic Disorders

A. *Primary:* Predictors of Neural Integrity
   1. *Age:* Greater recovery for younger than for older patients.
   2. *Etiology:* Patients with traumatic lesion have better expected recovery than patients with cerebrovascular accident.
   3. *Site of Lesion:* Greater recovery for patients with anterior compared to posterior dominant hemisphere lesion.
   4. *Extent of Lesion:* Better expected recovery for patients with small lesion compared to large lesion.
   5. *Handedness—Cerebral Dominance:* Left-handed and ambidextrous patients demonstrate greater recovery than do right-handed patients.

B. *Secondary:* Behavioral Characteristics Reflecting Neural Integrity
   1. *Aphasia Type:* Greater recovery for patients with Broca's aphasia than with Wernicke's or global aphasia.
   2. *Aphasia Severity:* Better recovery for mild than for severe aphasia.
   3. *Sensory and Motor Deficits:* More limited recovery when sensory and motor deficits are present.
   4. *Time Since Onset:* Early therapy intervention produces better recovery.

C. *Tertiary:* Psychosocial and Other Factors
   1. *Emotional Status:* Better recovery if patient recognizes and accepts deficits and is motivated to improve.
   2. *Residential Environment:* Patients in family setting demonstrate greater recovery than those in institutional facility.
   3. *Intelligence and Education:* Recovery greater for patients with superior intellectual abilities and higher levels of educational attainment.
   4. *Associated Medical Problems:* Presence of associated medical problems reduces level of expected recovery.

various neuromuscular and sensory deficits. *Tertiary* factors include motivation, education, and living environment, characteristics typically not directly related to the brain damage.

LaPointe (1978) provides a somewhat different classification. His system includes *subject variables* (age, education, intelligence, handedness), *medical variables* (etiology, site, and extent of lesion; associated medical problems), *speech-language variables* (type and severity of aphasia, coexisting motor speech impairment, sensory-perceptual deficits), and *other variables* (months since onset, motivation, emotional status, environment).

A qualification (or more aptly stated—a precaution) must precede the consideration of prognostic indicators. Neither the predictive value of a single variable nor group of variables is specifically known; multiple regressions have not been completed to provide such weightings. Therefore indicators cannot be strictly applied to the next aphasic patient examined in the clinic. They should be viewed as general guidelines rather than specific rules of operation.

primary prognostic indicators

Age Many studies agree that age is a potent negative prognostic indicator (Eisenson, 1949, 1964; Kertesz and McCabe, 1977; Sands, Sarno, and Shankweiler, 1969; Smith, 1971, 1972; Tikofsky, Kooi, and Thomas,

1960; Wepman, 1951). This holds true whether the lesion is of traumatic (Wepman, 1951) or cerebrovascular (Smith, 1972) origin. However research findings have not consistently borne out this observation. Culton (1971) found that when a group of ten subjects was divided at the median age the five best recovered patients were older (mean—55 years) than the five least improved (mean—48 years). In a previously discussed study, Deal and Deal (1978) found no significant correlations between age and overall Porch Index of Communicative Ability change scores and no significant differences between groups when the sample was divided into subjects more than and less than 55 years of age. The point to be made is that, although age is an important prognostic indicator, its effects cannot be considered independently of other factors, such as site, etiology, and extent of lesion.

Since the purpose here is to provide a rationale for use of prognostic indicators, some neurophysiological and neurostructural changes associated with aging need to be examined. Like other organs of the body, the brain undergoes structural changes with aging. Brain weight and neuronal population reduces, the cortical ribbon narrows, the sulci widen, the volume of the subarachnoid space increases and the ventricular system dilates (Brody, 1970). In a frequently cited study, Appel and Appel (1942a, 1942b) found that there was a linear regression in brain weight from maturity (25 years of age) that amounted to 11 percent of the mean brain weight by 96 years of age. Bondareff (1959) noted that brain volume relative to skull capacity decreased as a function of age.

Coupled to the reduction in brain weight are decreases in neuronal density. Brody (1955) examined the brains of 20 individuals between birth and 95 years who died from causes not expected to have an effect on cortical nerve cells. After examining the precentral and postcentral gyri, the superior and inferior temporal gyri, and the striate area, he found a significant negative correlation between cell counts and age. He also noted that the neuronal depopulation was not uniform; the greatest decrease from 20 to 95 years occurred in the superior temporal gyrus with less decrease in the postcentral area and visual cortex. The decrease in the postcentral area reduced cell counts to one-third of what would be expected at 19 years of age. In a later study of the superior frontal gyrus, Brody (1970) found the most marked reductions in cell counts in the fifth decade (40 to 50 years of age) with further decreases occurring at slower rates so that by the ninth decade (80 to 90 years of age) neurons were reduced by 50 percent.

Additional microscopic changes include an increase in senile plaques, accumulation of aging pigments, and formation of neurofibrillary tangles (Berry, 1975; Brody and Vyayashankar, 1977). The physiological bases of these changes are poorly understood.

The brain is functionally tied to the cerebrovascular system and the advent and advance of arteriosclerosis is expected to have an impact on neurological function. Since interruptions and reductions in blood supply produce neuronal death and cerebrovascular disease is primarily restricted to the elderly, age is expected to not only reduce the number of neurons but also to reduce the restitution of neuronal function. Smith (1971), for example, noted that the effects of diaschisis persist for a longer period of time following brain damage in the elderly and that the ability of tissue to recover and compensate for loss of function decreases with age.

Behavioral changes in normal aging will also have an impact on recovery whether they are due to neurophysiological and neurostructural changes or not. Normal elderly have been viewed as being more cautious and rigid in their behavior. These characteristics may be due to intellectual decline and a reduced ability to cope with complex problems (Miller, 1977). Part of the evidence for reduced intellectual ability of the aged derives from Wechsler's standardization of the Adult Intelligence Scale. More recent data (Schaie and Strother, 1968a, 1968b) suggests that the intellectual decline may not be as great as indicated by Wechsler's results and is more pronounced on performance than on verbal tasks.

In terms of problem solving, studies which have provided opportunities for subjects to elicit information showed that the aged make more inquiries, especially redundant noninformative inquiries. Additionally the elderly make less effective use of the information that they have requested or that has been presented by the experimenter. Their analysis (obtaining information) and synthesis (processing information to arrive at a solution) skills both seem to be impaired (Arenberg, 1973; Botwinick, 1970; Jerome, 1963; Wiersma and Klausmeier, 1965; Young, 1966).

Increased age is accompanied by reductions in memory (Barrett, 1972), although this is not a consistent effect. Botwinick (1967) pointed out that memory decline is descriptive of more and more individuals as they get older, although some elderly retain a relatively intact memory regardless of age. A distinction needs to be made between short- and long-term memory. Long-term memory, such as personal history, past experience, and knowledge, tends not to be lost with aging. Short-term memory for recently learned information, on the other hand, appears more susceptible to the effects of aging (Barrett, 1972; Kimmel, 1974). In a review of the literature, Craik (1977) concluded that only minimal changes in short-term memory occur with increasing age. However when the information to be remembered exceeds the capacity of the short-term store, older subjects have more difficulty. They have problems in both acquisition and retrieval, especially when tasks require divided attention, reorganization of information in memory, or use of mediation strategies. Craik attributed both acquisition and retrieval problems to a failure to engage in deep semantic processing of information.

In summary, reduced expected recovery as a function of age is due to neurological, cerebrovascular, and behavioral changes. The elderly patient is less capable of responding and compensating for neurological insult because the brain and cerebrovascular system have been at least partially compromised by aging. Moreover the behavioral processes necessary for communicative recovery, learning, memory, and problem solving have also been reduced to produce decreased ultimate expected level of communicative return of function.

Etiology The etiology of brain damage will aid in predicting rate and final level of recovery. It is generally recognized that a patient with a traumatically induced lesion will enjoy a better prognosis than will a patient with a cerebrovascular etiology. Moreover the course of recovery will vary as a function of the *type* of trauma or stroke. For example, Johnson (1975) compared the recovery patterns of five patients with subdural hematoma with five patients with intracerebral hematoma on the Porch Index of Communicative Ability, The course of recovery for the subdural hematoma patients was rapid and occurred within 8 to 12 weeks postoperatively; the recovery of the intracerebral patients was slow and, in general, required two years to reach performance levels equivalent to the subdural patients. Rubens (1977) observed that the recovery pattern of the patient with a hemorrhagic etiology may be delayed from up to three months or more when compared to patients with other types of cerebrovascular lesions.

Etiology is related to age. Younger aphasic patients more frequently have traumatic lesions, while older patients more typically have cerebrovascular etiologies. No studies have examined matched age groups of traumatic and stroke etiology patients. Most of the information on traumatic aphasics derives from investigations of young patients with war-related missile wounds (Russell and Espir, 1961; Wepman, 1951), while cerebrovascular etiology studies have primarily included older patients (Sands et al., 1969; Sarno and Levita, 1979; Sarno et al., 1970). For example, the traumatic group studied by Smith (1972) had a mean age of 27.9 years and the stroke group a mean age of 48.4 years. Wepman's traumatic patients had a mean age of 25.8 years; Sands et al.'s poststroke patients, 56.5 years.

The basic rationale for the inclusion of etiology as a prognostic indicator is that strokes typically occur on a backdrop of cerebrovascular disease. Since cerebrovascular disease is most commonly a consequence of aging, a direct prognostic relationship exists between the two factors. However insufficient data is available to systematically factor out the effects of age from that of etiology. What might be concluded is that, insofar as strokes reflect cerebrovascular integrity, they are predictive of recovery.

Site and Extent of Lesion In a study of a large number of wartime missile wound patients, Russell and Espir (1961) noted that the site and extent of brain damage were related to the severity and type of aphasia. It should be intuitively apparent that these two factors—site and extent of lesion—are prognostically significant. More brain damage generates a poorer prognosis than less brain damage, and damage to the primary cortical speech and language representation areas of the dominant hemisphere is more detrimental to recovery than lesions to neural structures peripheral or distant to these areas.

These observations are supported by the results of data-based investigation and clinical observation. Utilizing computerized transaxial brain scans, Yarnell, Monroe, and Sobel (1976) studied the relationship of size, location, and number of cerebral lesions to aphasia outcome in 14 patients with thromboembolic cerebrovascular insults. Recovery was determined by comparison of severity ratings derived from results of an aphasia test battery administered at one month and at a follow-up time which occurred from eight months to 3.5 years post-onset of brain damage, depending on the patient. Yarnell et al. found that large single lesions correlated with poorer recovery than did small single lesions and that bilateral lesions helped to account for significant residual aphasia. In terms of site of brain damage Eisenson (1964) observed that patients with single lesions to the temporoparietal area had a slower recovery than did patients with lesions outside of this area.

Handedness—Cerebral Dominance Handedness is a prognostic indicator insofar as it is reflective of cerebral dominance. In other words, left-handed and ambidextrous patients have a higher incidence of incompletely lateralized cerebral dominance, and the consequences of a dominant hemisphere lesion on linguistic processes are less acute although more frequent. In a clinical report of 161 aphasic patients with unilateral hemisphere lesions, Subirana (1958) observed, "The more an individual is basically right-handed the less we shall expect to see the regression of his aphasia" (p. 424). Based on a literature review and study of chronic aphasia, Smith (1971, 1972) concluded that ". . . although acute aphasia may occur more frequently in left- than right-handed adults with cerebral lesions, chronic aphasia is less frequent in sinistrals." Finally, in an investigation of 57 right-handed and 57 left-handed patients with almost identical lesions of one cerebral hemisphere verified postmortem, Gloning (1977) noted, among other findings, that aphasia occurred with left and right hemisphere damage in nonright-handed patients, and that the most transient aphasias were found in nonright-handed patients. What might be concluded then is that in nonright-handed patients the aphasia will be less severe and the recovery more rapid and more complete due to the bilateral representation of language.

secondary prognostic indicators

The primary indicators discussed so far relate specifically to the premorbid or post-onset status of the brain at the time of evaluation. A number of second-order parameters that are measurable behaviors inferen-

tially related to neural functioning also have been identified as prognostically significant.

Type and Extent of Aphasia It is generally agreed that aphasia
severity is a negative prognostic indicator. In a study of 70 cases, Butfield
and Zangwill (1946) found that the highest percentage of "marked improvement" (58 percent) occurred in mildly involved patients, and the lowest
percentage (40 percent) occurred in severely involved aphasics. Patients
were primarily young adults with traumatic lesions. Schuell et al. (1964)
observed that the poorest prognosis was for patients classified as demonstrating an irreversible aphasia syndrome characterized by almost a complete loss of functional language skills in all modalities. Sands et al. (1969)
found that the lower the level of performance at entrance to a rehabilitation
program, the poorer the prognosis for 30 patients studied. They concluded
that ". . . the severity of the language impairment at initial evaluation is a
moderately good predictor of the amount of recovery that can be expected"
(p. 205). In a study of 30 severely aphasic patients, Sarno, Silverman, and
Sands (1970) found no significant improvement in treated and untreated
patients and suggested that therapy did not modify verbal behavior in this
group. Several other investigators have documented poorer recovery for
severely involved aphasics (Godfrey, 1959; Godfrey and Douglass, 1959;
Kenin and Swisher, 1972; Kertesz and McCabe, 1977). It can be concluded,
then, that aphasia severity is directly related to recovery. However aphasia
severity cannot be considered independently of aphasia type.

In most studies of aphasia severity, patients are not classified by type of
disorder and then grouped according to severity. This type of grouping is
not practical, theoretical considerations notwithstanding, because aphasia
test batteries do not have subtests for comparable skills in different modalities that are of equal difficulty. The Porch Index of Communicative Abilities,
for example, has taken this into account, and performance is displayed as
a function of subtest difficulty. Severity is used as a prognostic indicator
based on group comparisons of different severity levels disregarding
aphasia type or inherent severity differences between groups.

Butfield and Zangwill (1946), Marks, Taylor, and Rusk (1957), and
Kertesz and McCabe (1977) reported that patients with an expressive
aphasia have a better prognosis for recovery than do patients with a global
aphasia. Lomas and Kertesz (1978) investigated 31 patients divided into
four groups (high fluency/high comprehension; high fluency/low comprehension; low fluency/high comprehension; low fluency/low comprehension) on the basis of fluency of spontaneous speech and auditory word
discrimination. Patients were tested within 30 days of onset and at three
months with the Western Aphasia Battery. None was treated between evaluations. Results revealed that the low fluency/low comprehension group
improved significantly less and the low fluency/high comprehension group

significantly more than the other three groups. Assuming that these two groups are indicative of global and Broca's aphasics, respectively, the results support the better prognosis for expressive aphasics.

Several points are relevant to the discussion of severity and type of aphasia as prognostic indicators. Neither is independent of site or extent of lesion nor of age—primary indicators related to the status of the brain. In a study previously reviewed, Yarnell et al. (1976) found that bilateral or large dominant hemisphere lesions correlated with global aphasia and generally poorer recovery, while relatively small dominant hemisphere lesions correlated with expressive, rather than receptive, deficits and a "more benign aphasia resolution" (p. 522). Obler et al. (1978) found that in 167 right-handed males with confirmed neurological lesions Broca's aphasics tended to be younger than any other type, while Wernicke's aphasics were significantly older than the average aphasic. Furthermore the incidence of Wernicke's aphasia increased with age while other types declined. Smith (1971) noted that patients with severe auditory comprehension deficits were older (51.9 years) than those with moderate (45.5 years) and mild (47.5 years) deficits.

What might be concluded is that Broca's aphasics have a better prognosis because they are younger and have more limited lesions, while Wernicke's and global aphasics are older and have more extensive brain damage. This conclusion addresses the issue of the status of the brain rather than differential prognoses based upon aphasia type because there is no data to answer this question. What seems apparent, however, is that marked recovery of communicative functioning requires auditory comprehension facility and that severe comprehension deficits suggest a poor prognosis for recovery (Brown, 1960; Schuell, 1955). Lomas and Kertesz (1978) observed that ". . . the initial level of comprehension may predict the extent of expressive language recovery. Only those groups initially high on comprehension showed appreciable improvements in expressive language" (p. 398). However this is not a universal finding. Sarno, Silverman, and Levita (1970) found that auditory comprehension was not significantly related to recovery, although all their patients were severely impaired in "understanding" on the Functional Communication Profile.

Finally, it should be pointed out that other aspects of the aphasia may be of prognostic significance. Wepman (1953) observed that the ability to recognize and correct errors was a positive prognostic sign. Additionally statistical procedures have been used to predict recovery at 3, 6, and 12 months post-onset by means of test results obtained at one month on the Porch Index of Communicative Ability (Porch, Wertz, and Collins, 1974).

Associated Sensory and Motor Deficits It has been proposed that the presence of sensory deficits has an adverse effect on recovery (Anderson, Bourestom, and Greenberg, 1970; Eisenson, 1964). The presence of hemiplegia is indicative of a greater initial language impairment, although hemiplegic and nonhemiplegic patients can benefit from therapy (Smith, 1972). A significantly poorer prognosis is predicted for patients with hemiplegia because there is a higher incidence of global aphasia, global aphasics with hemiplegia are older, and global hemiplegic patients demonstrate a higher incidence of sensory and severe comprehension deficits (Smith, 1972). Smith concluded that ". . . it is reasonable to assume that such defects (sensory defects) in hemiplegic aphasics generally indicate more extensive brain damage than in hemiplegic aphasics without sensory defects; and similarly, more extensive brain damage in nonhemiplegic aphasics with sensory defects" (p. 22).

A poorer prognosis for patients with sensory and motor deficits is predicated on their more extensive brain damage. It also is noteworthy that these deficits may serve as impediments to treatment and recovery in that they reduce sensory access and limit motor responses.

Time from Aphasia Onset to Initiation of Therapy There is an apparent consensus that early treatment post-onset of brain damage produces greater return of function than if therapy is initiated at a later time. This holds true whether comparisons are made between patients for whom therapy was begun within six months and more than six months (Butfield and Zangwill, 1946); within one year and more than one year (Wepman, 1951); less than two months, between two and six months, and more than six months (Basso et al., 1979; Vignolo, 1964); within two months and more than four months (Sands et al., 1969). When measured in terms of improved test scores, at least a portion of early treatment effects appears to be attributed to spontaneous recovery although Sands et al. (1969) observed, "Neither can we exclude the possibility that early treatment is advantageous" (p. 206). If recovery is significantly enhanced by early treatment, the neurophysiological bases for this time frame of increased therapy intervention effects have never been explained. Two hypotheses appear plausible, but neither is particularly tenable. The first has an analogy in the atrophic changes of muscle associated with disuse. Perhaps an extended period post-onset of brain damage with limited communication possible has the effect of producing atrophic changes in linguistic ability. A second possibility is that brain damage produces a newfound cortical plasticity analogous to periods in neural maturation during which language learning is optimized. At present there appears to be no data to account for enhanced treatment effects with early intervention.

tertiary prognostic indicators

Tertiary factors encompass premorbid characteristics of the patient, aspects of his or her environment, and concomitant medical conditions that may affect recovery. These factors are not directly related to the status of the brain. This does not mean that they are unimportant—they may have a marked impact on expected recovery.

Emotional Factors The emotional status of the patient may be critical to recovery. Eisenson (1949) observed, "The patient with an outgoing personality who is not given to doing much introspection, who is willing to take a chance on making a speech response even though the response may be a wrong one, is much more likely to improve to a point approximating his preinjury state than is a patient who is withdrawn, introspective and generally inhibited" (p. 263). Eisenson also noted that persistent euphoria, too high expectations of recovery, and overdependency were negative prognostic factors. The importance of acceptance and motivation cannot be underestimated. A refusal to recognize and accept communicative deficits and a lack of motivation to actively participate in communicative rehabilitation must be viewed as negative prognostic indicators.

Residential Environment (Social Milieu) The effects of the patient's living environment have not been investigated. Patients residing in a nursing facility would be expected to have more severe deficits, and more difficulty caring for themselves independently; therefore, their prognosis would be expected to be poorer. The only study that has specifically examined environmental factors in recovery (Sarno, Silverman, and Levita, 1970) found no significant difference in recovery between patients residing at home, in a nursing home, or in a hospital or rehabilitation center. Although the importance of the living environment has been stressed (Eisenson, 1964; Schuell et al., 1964), its prognostic significance has not been established.

Intelligence and Education Darley (1972) observed that patients with higher intelligence make greater gains in therapy, a conclusion tentatively agreed upon by Eisenson (1973). A comparable statement might be appropriate for the effects of education since a positive relationship would be expected between intelligence and education. Evidence to date is fragmentary (Sarno, Silverman, and Levita, 1970; Wepman, 1951) and a definitive statement is not possible. However the conclusions of Eisenson seem appropriate: "On the whole . . . prognosis is more favorable for persons at the upper end of the intelligence scale and for the highly educated than for those at the low end of the scale" (p. 124).

○ PROGNOSES FOR OTHER ACQUIRED
  NEUROGENIC DISORDERS

Apraxia The prognosis for apraxia is determined on most of the same variables as have been discussed for aphasia. In fact, most of the studies reviewed did not make distinctions between aphasia and apraxia since verbal apraxia is most frequently viewed as a primary characteristic of Broca's aphasia. Wertz (1978), however, reviewed studies pertinent to prognosis in apraxia (e.g., Butfield and Zangwill, 1946; Vignolo, 1964; Webb and Love, 1974) and concluded that ". . . the patient without coexisting oral-nonverbal apraxia, a short duration, mild-to-moderate severity, minimal coexisting aphasia, and demonstrated learning and generalization has a better prognosis for recovery than apraxic patients displaying the converse of each feature" (p. 70).

Dysarthria, Language of Confusion, Language of Generalized Intellectual Deterioration No efficacy or prognosis studies have been completed for dysarthria, confusion, or dementia. A primary difference between these disorders and aphasia and apraxia is that the former are more variable because the neurological conditions from which they evolve are frequently progressive or are characterized by remissions associated with the disease process or the medical treatment applied. In general, the same prognostic factors are considered: status of the nervous system, behavioral correlates of brain damage, and emotional-environmental aspects of the patient.

At this point a return to the five patients described in Chapter Two would be fruitful in demonstrating application of prognostic indicators. These patients served as examples for evaluation procedures. As used here, prognosis denotes the extent to which recovery approaches premorbid communication abilities. Normal function therefore is used as the reference in contrast to more limited references like development of a nonoral alternative communication system or reacquisition of third-grade-level reading skills.

A case summary will be presented for each patient. Based on this available data, a prognostic statement will be decided upon. A five-point scale will be used (very poor, poor, fair, good, excellent). The indicators and prognosis for each of the patients is presented in Table 3–3.

Patient J., a 63-year-old right-handed vocational counselor, suffered a small left occipital infarct with alexia and right homonymous hemianopsia. She also demonstrated cognitive decline typically associated with diffuse cortical degeneration. J. was unmarried and lived with a housekeeper. Education, intelligence, and vocational attainment were considered above average premorbidly. She was highly motivated to improve communicative functioning through therapy. However her judgment was impaired, and she was unwilling to accept the severity of the problem or the limitations it imposed on her activity. The prognosis for recovery was very poor. The primary reason for this decision is the presence of progressive cortical degeneration which would be expected to severely compromise any benefits of therapy.

Patient B., a 16-year-old right-handed high school student suffered a small parietal-occipital area stab wound with anomia and right homonymous

TABLE 3–3

Prognosis for Recovery of Communicative Abilities in Five Patients with Neurogenic Disorders

VARIABLE	PATIENT				
	J.	*B.*	*P.*	*C.*	*S.*
Age	–	+	+	+	–
Etiology	–	+	–	–	–
Site	–	–	–	o	o
Extent	–	+	–	o	–
Handedness	+	+	+	o	o
Disorder Type	–	+	–	o	–
Disorder Severity	–	+	–	o	o
Associated Deficits	o	o	–	o	o
Time from Onset to Treatment	+	+	+	+	o
Emotional Status	–	+	–	+	+
Environment	+	+	–	+	+
Intelligence Education	+	o	–	+	+
Associated Medical Problems	+	+	–	+	–
PROGNOSIS	Very Poor	Good	Poor	Good	Poor

Key: + positive
    – negative
    o not applicable, undetermined, or equivocal

hemianopsia. He was one of ten children residing at home with his father, a tile layer, and mother, a housewife. The family moved frequently, and the patient was disruptive in school. He was motivated to engage in treatment for his communicative handicap. Due to the type and limited extent of brain damage, age and motivation of the patient, and lack of medical complications, the prognosis for recovery was considered good. Given a more stable emotional makeup and home environment, prognosis would be excellent.

Patient P., a 34-year-old right-handed housewife, was referred with stroke syndrome following strep meningitis of the entire left hemisphere. Evaluation revealed a severe aphasia. Sensory and motor deficits included right hemiplegia, hemianesthesia, homonymous hemianopsia, and facial weakness. The patient was married to a custodian and had not completed high school. She was the mother of four children and suffered from severe diabetes controlled with insulin. The home situation was unstable. Two children had quit high school, and the family had not adjusted to the altered role of the patient. P. was not highly motivated in seeking or attending therapy. The prognosis for her was rated as poor due to the extent of brain damage, severity of the aphasia, associated medical problems, sensory and motor deficits, and the unstable home situation.

Patient C., a 49-year-old retired airline pilot, suffered a bilateral medullary infarct with moderate flaccid dysarthria. Motor impairment included quadriparesis and weakness of the oral-facial musculature. The major sensory deficit was a moderate bilateral sensorineural hearing loss. No cognitive or language deficits were noted. He was a college-educated widowed father of three children and was highly motivated and goal directed. There was no history of other major medical problems. Prognosis for recovery was judged to be good based on age, limited lesion size, moderate speech deficit, and psychosocial factors.

Patient S., a 62-year-old college professor with Parkinson's disease, demonstrated a moderate hypokinetic dysarthria. Associated medical problems included ulcers and congestive heart disease. Intellectual ability and education were superior. The patient was married, lived at home, and was highly motivated to improve communicative functioning so that he could return to the classroom. Based on the progressive nature of the neurological disease and associated medical problems, prognosis for recovery of function was poor.

SUMMARY

Rehabilitation cannot be efficiently carried out without consideration of three factors: physiological aspects of recovery, the value of the treatment applied, and the variables that will allow a prediction of treatment outcome. The most important of the three is the determination of prognosis—but it cannot be arrived at accurately without knowledge of the other two areas discussed. A determination of which patient has the best prognosis is not possible by mathematical computation. The factors must be individually weighed, and a judgment made. There is no assurance that the prediction will always be right. The clinician's responsibility is not always to be right; rather it is to make the best judgment possible and to be willing to change an opinion if the patient's situation warrants it. No factor weightings for prognosis have been provided because it is not known whether a young severely involved aphasic has a better prognosis than an elderly mildly involved aphasic, whether the effects of brain tissue loss are more important than the patient's motivation, or any other combination of factors that need to be considered. What has been pointed out are the variables that need to be identified and a rationale for the importance of each in determining (predicting) treatment outcome.

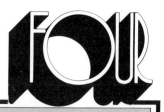

FOUR

Therapy form and content

○ INTRODUCTION

Therapy forms are defined here as the structured rationales that give rise to specific therapeutic procedures and modes of operation. *Therapy content,* in contrast, is the collection of stimuli placed in the scaffolding of therapy forms to address specific communicative deficits. In general, no clear distinctions can be made between different forms or between forms and content. Both forms and content may change and, in fact, must be reasonably plastic in order to accommodate the needs of individual patients. The specific therapeutic needs of patients may be the major reason why replicable procedures for the treatment of a single patient do not exist in published form. There are case studies of treatment methods, established principles of therapy, and rationales for procedures used but no description of the exact methodology encompassed in the complete treatment of a patient. It must be recognized, then, that the following discussion will not provide an exacting prescription of how to treat the next patient referred.

Therapy approaches are not—or at least should not be—developed serendipitously. They should be founded on well-established principles and knowledge of the patient and the disorder. The importance of benefits accruing to patients from procedures that have resulted from trial and error should not be denied, but these procedures should not be determined by happenstance and are enhanced and more efficient if developed from a known data base. As part of the discussion, evidence supportive of particular approaches to treatment will be considered since it is an important determinant of the quality of the methodology.

This chapter is divided into four sections. The first and largest section deals with treatment emphasizing rehabilitation of speech and language. Ideally, the purpose of these therapy approaches is to reestablish speech and language to premorbid levels of functioning. Included are a review of therapy rationales, stimulus attributes and presentation procedures, and specific treatment methods. The specific methods reviewed are not an exhaustive listing and are not presented in sufficient detail, in most cases, to allow immediate clinical application, but provide a cross-section of those available for the treatment of neurogenic patients. Second, nonverbal communication techniques are considered. Since some neurogenic patients are not capable of developing oral communication, other modes must have an important focus is the discussion of therapy forms and content. Third, treatment which emphasizes improving the efficiency of communicative interaction between the patient and speaking partner are discussed. These methods are concerned with capitalizing on the compensatory strategies and residual speech and language skills of the patient in order to maximize communication success. Finally, group therapy, which has been used for speech and language rehabilitation, socialization, and psychotherapy, is considered.

○ THERAPY EMPHASIZING REHABILITATION OF SPEECH AND LANGUAGE
RATIONALES

stimulation approach to treatment

The stimulation approach to therapy was originally described by Wepman (1947, 1951, 1953) and formalized by Schuell and associates (Schuell, Carroll, and Street, 1955; Schuell et al., 1964). Basically, this approach is predicated on the notion that aphasia is an interference with, rather than a loss of, function and that sensory stimulation may aid in reducing disrupted communicative processes. It is not based, then, on learning principles per se, although learning certainly occurs as part of the treatment, but rather on the assumption that sensory stimulation aids in reestablishing cortical integrations. Wepman (1951) observed:

> ... it is held ... that aphasia is a disorder affecting the patient's *total reaction pattern* due to a disturbance of the integrating capacity of the cortex. This working theory stresses the necessity for considering the patient as an individual in need of reestablishing the use of neural capacities which are present and potentially functional, but which are blocked from use by the pathological condition existing within the cortex (pp. 85–86). . . . (consequently) aphasia therapy should not be conceived as a simple process of developing a new vocabulary or of adding newly learned language concepts. Rather, it must be a process of assisting the patient through a variety of stimulations in his groping toward ego-integrity through new cortical integrations by his remaining motor cortex. (p. 263)

Wepman proposed that during the primary stage of recovery therapy takes the form of naming environmental objects for the patient without expectation of a response. No great import is assigned to the particular nouns chosen since the purpose is to integrate cerebral mechanisms rather than to generate specific learning by stimulus-response drill. What is important is that the words selected be appropriate and that the stimuli provided be repetitive. Presentation and naming of the object may be supplemented by additional cues such as demonstrating the use of the object or graphically displaying in written form the name of the object. The patient's response is not evaluated for accuracy, and the therapist's continual approval of every effort is a rule of thumb. After naming is established, verbs, adjectives, and adverbs are added to produce short telegraphic sentences. Reading and writing activities are introduced at an early point in the program to supplement the auditory stimulation provided.

Wepman (1953) later conceptualized the stimulation method according to three parameters on which aphasic patients could be considered: stimulation, facilitation, and motivation. He noted that patients differed in their ability to be stimulated but that the particular therapy procedures did not appear to matter since patients ". . . seem to get better or do not get better in approximately the same proportions, regardless of the approach used with them . . . [and therefore] the content of our therapy is of less importance than the manner in which it is conducted" (p. 6). *Facilitation* was defined as the physiological readiness of the patient to respond to stimulation and thereby reestablish cortical integrations. This conceptualization of stimulation and facilitation has an important analogy in neuronal excitability.

When a neuron receives an adequate (suprathreshold) stimulus, an action potential is developed which travels from cell body to axon. Although its function might be viewed as "all-or-none" (the stimulus is either adequate or inadequate to generate an action potential), the presence of inhibitory and facilitatory synapses between neurons and within neuronal chains produces functional plasticity. Pools of neurons repetitively fired are thought to become progressively more available for use. In this analogy facilitation relates to the relative excitability of neurons and neuronal chains—that is, their relative responsiveness to stimuli and, in Wepman's conceptualization, to the physiological readiness of the patient to respond. The intensity of stimulation required to generate a response would be affected by facilitatory and inhibitory influences operating on the neuronal chain or, in the case of the patient, the physiological, psychological, and emotional factors that affect receptivity to stimulation. Consequently the neurons or the patient may require various stimulus intensity gradations in order to respond. In some cases a response may not be induced by any intensity of the stimulus. With repeated stimulation at times the neuronal chain or patient is in a physiological state of readiness to respond, integrations occur which become progressively more accessible for use. One primary effect on this process, and the third parameter of Wepman's construct, is *motivation* which would be expected to govern the responsiveness of the patient.

The simple analogy between the stimulation approach and neuronal function was not proposed by Wepman but certainly follows his conceptualization of this approach:

> Aphasia therapy reduced to its primary function becomes . . . a process by which the therapist provides stimulative material in the area of the patient's

greatest need at a time when the nervous system is capable of utilizing it for the facilitation of cortical integrations leading to language performance (p. 12).

Wepman's formulation of stimulation therapy was given additional structure and specificity by Schuell (Jenkins, Jiminez-Pabon, Shaw, and Sefer, 1975). She observed that the clinician's task was ". . . to communicate with the patient and to stimulate disrupted processes to function maximally." she proposed seven principles of treatment:

1. Intensive auditory stimulation should be used but not alone since other sensory modalities may allow facilitation of a response.
2. The stimulus must be adequate to get into the brain and may need to be manipulated to produce a response.
3. Repetitive sensory stimulation should be provided.
4. Each stimulus should elicit a response so that the clinician can determine the adequacy of the stimulus and the patient can benefit from feedback available from the response.
5. Responses should be elicited, not forced.
6. The clinician should stimulate rather than correct responses.
7. One language modality should be used to facilitate another.

Wepman (1951), Schuell et al (1955), and Jenkins et al. (1975) provide some examples of therapy materials and procedures, but stimulation therapy for aphasia would seem to have taken many forms. Taylor (1964) reviewed some of the many adaptations of this approach and divided them into two overlapping categories: (1) nonspecific stimulation approaches and (2) specific stimulation approaches. The nonspecific approaches included the following:

1. *Spontaneous Recovery Approach.* This approach does not include therapy at all but simply monitors gains that can be attributed to physiological recovery.
2. *Environmental Stimulation Approach.* During the recovery period the patient is bombarded with verbal stimulation by individuals in the environment, including hospital staff, family, and friends.
3. *Rapport Approach.* A warm relationship is developed between the patient and clinician which serves as the vehicle for improved function regardless of therapy method or content.
4. *Socialization Approach.* Group activities, including singing and conversation, are the basis for increased motivation and communicative interaction.
5. *Psychotherapeutic Approach.* Individual or group settings are arranged in which the psychological and emotional concomitants of brain damage, such as anxiety, frustration, or anger, can be aired.

   6. *Interest Approach.* Lexical items of particular interest to the patient are selected and serve as the materials for the therapy sessions.

When viewed together these approaches appear to be helpful to the
patient by providing intense and varied environmental verbal stimulation,
a warm working relationship with the clinician, socialization with other
patients having similar problems so that emotional reactions to the disorder
can be discussed, and some input as to the types of stimuli to be used in
therapy sessions. The problem with these nonspecific techniques, however,
is that they have been used as the entire format for treatment rather than
as considerations in therapy planning.

The specific stimulation approaches included:

   1. *Association Approach.* Semantic units such as body parts, foods, clothing,
   and furniture, are chosen, and lexical items are placed in various contexts
   utilizing combinations of modalities. A word may be presented auditorily and
   the patient asked to repeat, copy, and read it. When the vocabulary items are
   established, they may be placed in contextual frames, such as *I bake a cake,
   I eat cake, please pass the cake,* and the procedure repeated with other
   vocabulary items in the module. The basic rationale is that the repeated
   contextual presentation and use of the word will strengthen associations and
   thereby become more readily accessible for the patient.

   2. *Situational Approach.* Everyday situations are constructed that will facilitate
   the learning of functional situational responses not ordinarily encompassed in
   task-oriented therapy. The approach is predicated on the observation that
   communication is less impaired than language and that the patient may utilize
   compensatory strategies, such as gestures, to communicate.

   3. *Auditory Stimulation Approach.* Relatively exclusive use of auditory stimulation serves as the basis of treatment on the premise that, since language is
   acquired primarily through audition, it will be the most effective means of
   reestablishing auditory comprehension, reading, writing, and verbal expression.

   4. *Minimal Differences Approach.* Orthographically and auditorily similar words
   serve as therapy material because of the belief that the aphasic patient's
   primary deficits lie in the inability to recognize minimal differences in language
   units.

It is obvious that the nonspecific and specific approaches reviewed by
Taylor significantly overlap; vary in scope, format, and content; and, in
some cases, do not bear a strong resemblance to the more task-oriented
procedures of Wepman and Schuell. Stimulation approaches have been
developed more recently which appear to vary somewhat from the rationale
that a stimulus presented when the patient is in a physiological readiness to
respond produces the cortical integrations necessary for language use.
However programmed instruction will be examined first.

programmed instruction approach to treatment

Programmed instruction is based on the rationale that aphasia results from a loss of brain tissue and with it a loss of acquired function and specific information. Therapy then takes the form of an educative process involving learning principles.

Learning in Aphasia　A number of studies have investigated learning in aphasia (Carson, Carson, and Tikofsky, 1968; Katz, 1958; Tikofsky, 1971;) Carson et al., for example, attempted to determine learning characteristics of aphasics and to establish stable differences in learning between normal and aphasic subjects. The performance of 64 aphasics and 64 normals on four types of experiments (stimulus uncertainty and response time, rote serial learning, repeated digit symbol task, rule learning task) was compared. Carson et al. found that the aphasics showed significant regularities in their ability to learn new tasks, to retain learned skills over time, and to handle a wide range of complexity of stimulus materials. Characteristics which distinguished them from normals were their slower speed and frequently their lower level of attainment. They did not differ from normals in their inability to perform on any of the difficult experimental tasks.

Several investigators (Filby and Edwards, 1963; Lane and Moore, 1962; Rosenberg, 1965; Rosenberg and Edwards, 1964, 1965) suggested that language dysfunction following brain damage may be viewed productively in terms of deficits in perceptual discrimination skills. Rosenberg, (1965) for example, assessed and trained in automated fashion perceptual discriminations which she believed were basic to reading. Five training programs utilized forms abstracted as those necessary to compose the symbols of the alphabet and were employed in shape, up-down, and right-left discrimination tasks. A verbal transfer test was composed of words, nonsense syllables, and individual letters. Data from the aphasic patients indicated that the training programs were effective in improving the latency of the discrimination response and that the improvement was demonstrated in transfer to verbal test items. Similarly Lane and Moore (1962) developed a consonant discrimination between /t/ and /d/ in an aphasic patient using spectrographic patterns and a pattern playback device.

In general, these studies, most of which used programmed instruction, demonstrate that learning in aphasic patients is dependable and progressive, that learned skills are retained, and that materials may vary over a wide range of complexity. However, learning would be expected to occur at a reduced rate and the final level of attainment is reduced when compared to normal subjects. With this in mind, parameters of the programmed instruction-behavior modification approach to treatment will be considered.

Brookshire (1967) has provided a description of the procedures entailed in programmed instruction. These include:

1. *Establishment of a Baseline.* The measurement of behaviors before treatment serve as the reference for determining treatment effects. The behaviors must be observable and reliably measurable. If not described in sufficient detail, changes in these behaviors may not be attributable to the treatment applied. The specific situation in which the behavior is measured must also be defined since the emission of responses is affected by the stimulus environment in which it occurs. Brookshire noted that the establishment of a stable baseline has the advantage of requiring that specific observable behaviors are defined before therapy is begun, including ". . . (a) the specific characteristics of the response of concern, (b) the stimulus situations which control the emission of the response of concern, (c) how consistently those stimulus situations cause the response to be emitted, and (d) how frequently the response of concern is emitted in each situation" (p. 22). A second advantage is that it provides a precise measure of the pretreatment behavior to be addressed so that responses during treatment can be compared to determine progress. This allows a culling out of those treatment procedures that do not generate progress toward a specified terminal goal and allows the maintenance of a high level of clinical efficiency.

2. *Application of Behavior Modification-Operant Conditioning Procedures.* Following establishment of a baseline, modification of the patient's behavior is initiated. This may involve either a change in the rate at which the response is emitted (such as increasing the frequency of correctly read single words) or the establishment of new responses. Both require that a precise description of the terminal behavior be developed. Change in the rate of responding basically involves structuring the stimulus situation so that the behavior of interest is emitted and then immediately reinforced or punished to increase or decrease its frequency. If a new response is to be developed, the behaviors of the patient must be carefully examined to find which ones have characteristics in common with the terminal behavior desired. Then successive approximations are used to shape the behavior. This will be produced by reinforcing those responses that are importantly similar to the terminal behavior. Initially responses are reinforced whenever they contain characteristics in common with the terminal behavior, but the limits of what constitutes reinforceable responses are gradually narrowed until the desired response is obtained. Thereafter only the terminal behavior is reinforced. In some cases responses are chained so that only the last element in a sequence of responses is reinforced and then only if the preceding responses are also observed. Thus the development of a response is based upon the existence of previous responses already conditioned.

3. *Extension of Stimulus Control.* Behaviors are emitted within specific stimulus environments, but at times they may be observable in only limited contexts when extension to other situations is wanted. The process of carry-over to other stimulus environments is accomplished by finding a stimulus situation in which the appropriate behavior is emitted. While reinforcing these responses, the stimulus context is systematically altered so that the behaviors are now observable in situations where previously they were not emitted. Coupled to the establishment of stimulus control may be changes in the reinforcement schedule so that they more closely approximate schedules (or lack thereof) in more commonly encountered communicative situations.

In summary, programmed instruction is made up of several chronological steps: (1) measurement of baseline response levels, (2) specification of the terminal behavior desired, (3) development of carefully controlled sequenced materials increasing in difficulty. These will ultimately yield the criterion or terminal behavior specified with empirically determined reinforcement of appropriate behaviors in order to increase the frequency of responding, to shape new behaviors, and/or to bring responses under stimulus control.

Operative principles of behavior modification are that a behavior must occur in order for a consequence to be applied, that many stimuli may control a single response, and that many consequences may govern a given behavior. In the typical clinical setting the variables to be dealt with in applying behavioral principles are the stimulus (antecedent event), the response, and the reinforcement (consequent event). Considerable attention has been given to programmed instruction in speech pathology (e.g., Costello, 1977) and specifically to the antecedent event (e.g., Hedrick, Christman, and Augustine, 1973) and consequent event (e.g., McReynolds, 1970). However aphasia therapy has not received much of this research interest (La Pointe, 1978).

The Antecedent Event   Attention to the antecedent event is important for two reasons. First, it significantly affects carry-over of learned behaviors to other communicative environments—that is, behaviors are maintained in varying situations by systematic attention to stimulus control. Second, it is assumed that the antecedent event (stimuli) necessary to elicit or facilitate the desired responses are hierarchically arranged by means of attributes of the stimuli and the cuing strategies used. One approach to treatment of aphasia which addresses attributes of the stimulus is Response Contingent Small-Step Treatment (RCSST) (Bollinger and Stout, 1976).

The RCSST entails consideration of the characteristics of the antecedent events necessary to elicit or cue a response. The task hierarchy is determined by the power (number of input modalities used, size or intensity of the stimulus, number of repetitions of the stimulus) of the antecedent and the number of choices and items per task in the stimulus-response field. The progression at each step of the program is from powerful stimuli and few choices in the response field to reductions of stimulus power and increases in response field choices.

The Consequent Event   In the clinical setting the patient's response is typically followed by a verbal "yes" or "no" contingency. However other types of consequences and their application have been investigated in aphasia. Studies have demonstrated that a delay in reinforcement may reduce performance (Brookshire, 1971a); that modeling and tokens, verbal compliments, correct response repetition, and objective feedback as reinforcers increase desired responses while punishment in the form of tokens and indications of the type of error decrease undesirable responses (Goodkin, 1966); and that punishment (time-out, response-cost, presentation of an aversive stimulus), although differentially effective, produces learning (Kushner, Hubbard, and Knox, 1973). Learning, however, is more rapid when positive reinforcement is combined with punishment.

It is usually sufficient in aphasia therapy to utilize a positive or negative verbal consequent event. Tangible positive reinforcers may be considered, but they may seem demeaning and become disparaging for the patient since improved communicative performance is a sufficient reward. Usually immediate and readily applicable contingencies, such as positive and negative verbal consequences, are sufficient for the motivated patient.

The Programs   Several studies have investigated the development and application of programmed instruction for aphasic patients. Taylor (1964) described a series of preverbal programs—nonverbal in the sense that no terminal behaviors were defined for reading, writing, oral expression, or auditory comprehension. Programs included activities such as imitation of body movements, matching and selecting like and unlike stimuli, and tracing and copying geometric forms. No oral-aural interaction was permitted during conduction of the sequences. Programs included a large number of steps administered by clinicians or on teaching machines, and requirements in terms of item administration and order were rigorously enforced. The total number of steps of the complete program was more than 5,000 encompassed within 20 individual teaching sequences. Taylor observed that the results of the pilot program were very encouraging. Patients who had not improved as a function of other techniques not only mastered the preverbal programs but also proceeded to acquire increased auditory comprehension and oral expressive skills. She also noted that, although the materials appeared monotonous, the patients were attentive, demonstrated markedly reduced anxiety, and appeared to exhibit less fatigue.

The advantages of programmed instruction were stated as follows:

> . . . (1) enables patient to work at his own rate of language learning; (2) has built-in measurements of language learning; (3) forces the clinician to work at patient's real level of functioning; (4) has built-in systematic record of responses to act as feedback for programming; (5) forces us to analyze terminal behaviors and appropriately design materials and methods for their realization; and (6) forces and facilitates a markedly increased precision in the description of language recovery for charts, progress notes, research and so forth. (p. 155)

Disadvantages cited included the observation that speech pathologists do not like programmed instruction because it reduces creativity and teaching sequences require a great deal of expense, planning, and analysis.

Programmed instruction as a vehicle for recovery from aphasia was also investigated by Holland and associates. Eighteen patients were included in the study (Holland, 1971), and seven were reported (Holland, 1970) to demonstrate the number and variety of the programs and to illustrate clinical considerations in programmed instruction. Table 4–1 shows the areas for which programs were written, the stimulus materials, and the requested responses. It was hoped that a group of programs could be developed which would serve as a core for working with aphasic patients in general, but this was not the case due to the heterogeneity of the patients studied. Consequently therapy planning for aphasia will always entail a certain amount of individualization.

TABLE 4–1

Summary of Programmed Approaches for Individual Patients

ACTIVITY	STIMULUS MODE	RESPONSE FORM
associational cuing	graphic, auditory	write, say
scrambled sentences	graphic	rearrange, write, and read aloud
sentence drills	graphic, auditory, pictures	write, say, read aloud, repeat
repetition	auditory	repeat
auditory memory	auditory	repeat
visual retention	objects	delayed naming
verb tense usage	graphic, auditory	write, say, choose from alternatives
active sentence usage	graphic, auditory, pictures	read aloud, repeat, say, write
job or interest-related word finding	graphic, auditory	say, write
dysarthria	auditory	repeat
scrambled transformations	graphic	rearrange, repeat
prepositions	pictures, graphic, objects	write
yes-no questions	auditory, graphic	say
written single words	graphic	trace-copy-write
simple reading comprehension	reading	answer questions
commands	auditory and common objects	follow instructions (nonverbal)
not	common objects and auditory	follow instructions (nonverbal)
adjective comprehension	written, auditory	final correct visual match
spelling (Bloomfield approach)	auditory	write
programmed editing	graphic	correct, write
scrambled words	graphic	match-to-sample, choose correct from alternatives

From Holland, A. Case studies in aphasia rehabilitation using programmed instruction. *J. Speech Hearing Dis.*, 1970, *35*, 377–390. Reprinted by permission.

Advantages of programmed instruction cited (Holland and Harris, 1968) included:

1. It allows measurement of treatment effects.
2. The patient's performance provides an analysis of how training occurs.
3. The patient as well as the clinician can observe progress, a powerful reinforcer.
4. Preparation of programs can be economical since there is a possibility they could be used with other patients.
5. The patient and the clinician are aware beforehand of what direction the program (therapy) will take, and the clinician is free to observe the patient and the therapy.

Programmed instruction has been found to be particularly adaptable to machine use (Keenan, 1966; Sarno, Silverman, and Sands, 1970) although personal clinical interaction also would be expected to improve the reinforcement chosen (Holland, 1970). At the same time the approach has been criticized because it has not completely considered the communicative disorders to be addressed.

In a review of major therapy approaches to aphasia, Seron, Van der Linden, and Van der Kaa-Delvenne (1978) made a distinction between structural and functional analyses of aphasia. Structural analyses deal with behavioral typography and are tied up with describing the modalities of impairment and verbal alterations characteristic of aphasia. Functional analyses, on the other hand, are used to define the conditions of communicative interaction and modifications of these activities in the aphasic patient. In an operant view,

> . . . functional analysis deals with all the contingencies which control acquisition and maintenance of verbal activity. Investigation of these contingencies involves systematic study of the relations between the stimuli which control speech production behavior, the verbal behavior itself, and the reinforcing consequences linked to speech production. (p. 78)

Seron et al. indicated that operant theory is capable of developing a sufficient functional analysis but so far has not considered structural analysis in detail.

In a critique of studies utilizing operant clinical procedures, they observed that the investigation of Sarno, Silverman, and Sands (1970) was insufficient because it (1) did not include a precise description (structural analysis) of the verbal behaviors of the global aphasic patients studied, (2) used reinforcement (presentation of correct response when error was made) that was less potent than the social reinforcers typical of verbal interaction, and (3) did not fully capitalize on motivation when it is remembered that the patients were faced with working through a possible total of more than 2,000 items in order to develop the use of a limited vocabulary. The clinical procedures of Holland were viewed as more valuable because individualization of treatment was observed, content was directed to the patient's interests, and clinician-patient interaction was allowed for some of the programs. However even with the institution of procedures of this type, Seron et al. observed that the primary goal of therapy should be the structuring of communicative situations in which verbal interaction occurs normally.

Programmed instruction has proven an intriguing approach to treatment, not only because of its adaptability to many types of communicative disorders and the ease with which it can be presented by machine, but also because it is replicable and thereby lends accountability to the therapy implemented. At the same time behavior modification has been somewhat disappointing (1) because a large proportion of the research has been directed toward skills identified as prerequisite to language rather than language itself and (2) because so little attention has been spent on gradual progression to a more comprehensive specification of language (Holland, 1975).

So far behavior modification and stimulation therapy have been viewed as having two distinct rationales when, in fact, almost any effective clinical strategy engenders facets of both their methodologies. Holland (1970) noted some similarities between the two: Programs can control the amount of stimulation, they can require continuous responding by the aphasic, they allow for restimulation, and they can continually be used to evaluate performance. Martin (1975) attempted to obviate the need for distinctions between the methods by identifying areas of common rationale. He observed that two basic assumptions—reductionism and peripheralism—underlie aphasia therapy and programmed instruction in particular. *Reductionism* is the process of breaking down a complex phenomenon into its basic components. This assumes that language is simply composed of units (phonemes) which are combined into larger units (words) to produce utterances. Reductionism suffers from two shortcomings: complexity is determined by the number of units, and a hierarchical arrangement of stimuli must be established and learned for the behavior to be reconstituted. The problem here is one of application rather than theory. Systems used to foster language analysis in themselves are artificial and, although they are critical for description, do not establish the hierarchy or ordering of language acquisition. *Peripheralism* is the effort to describe psychological processes as stimulus-response linkings between receptor and effector systems. It turns out to be an oversimplification of the complexities involved in aphasic language. A major identified shortcoming of stimulation approaches was the lack of an established rationale for the processes underlying therapy-derived recovery. Martin concluded that the approaches both were based on learning but different theories of learning—programmed instruction on a connectivist theory and stimulation therapy on cognitive theory.

Tied up with the stimulation and programmed instruction approaches are concepts which need to be considered further—*stimulation* and *facilitation.* Definitions must underlie description of these variables since their meaning is, at least to a small extent, at variance with the mixture of behavioral and physiological terms used earlier by Wepman. *Stimulation* is described as all aspects of the clinical environment controlled by the clinician and includes such parameters as saliency, context, and relationship between stimulus presentation and response. *Facilitation* is defined as what the patient does to produce an appropriate response and includes behaviors such as associated motor activities. This description of facilitation is different from that proposed by Wertz (1978) who defined it as ". . . an aid the clinician uses to increase the probability of a correct response [including, for example] stimulus repetition, cues, combining stimulus modes, and reducing the number of alternatives present in the task" (p. 31). Clearly these are aspects of the stimulus situation and not of the patient's efforts to respond.

○ THE STIMULUS

Characteristics of the stimulus are of importance to the ability of the patient to respond. This is true for all modalities of input, although the general consensus is that auditory input is most important in stimulation therapy. It is assumed that parameters of the stimulus can be hierarchically arranged to produce a level of responding that is not only continual but also correct (appropriate) more than half the time. It is also assumed that parameters contributing to the saliency of the stimulus and thereby increasing the probability of a correct response can be independently varied. It will not be the purpose here to review all the studies that provide the underpinnings for knowledge of stimulus attributes, context, and presentation since they are reviewed elsewhere (Darley, 1976; Duffy, 1981) but to summarize the more important findings.

Stimulus Attributes   Assuming some consistency from modality to modality (Goodglass, Barton, and Kaplan, 1968), increasing the probability of a correct response rests firmly on factors that enhance its magnitude. Magnitude can be described in terms of size, intensity, redundancy, operativity, complexity, and meaningfulness. Much available information on parameters of the stimulus that add to its magnitude has evolved from studies of naming and noun recognition. Although not a universal finding (e.g., Corlew and Nation, 1975), Visual stimuli that are large and unambiguous, and auditory stimuli presented at moderate intensity levels without background noise would be expected to have the greatest magnitude. Moreover their ability to elicit a correct response are enhanced by frequency of occurrence and meaningfulness—high frequency words of low abstraction level would most likely be effective (Spreen, 1968). Length of the stimulus also has an impact on the ability to elicit a correct response. Short words improve comprehension and production accuracy. Finally manipulable stimuli or pictures of manipulable stimuli appear to produce better performance.

Syntactic and Semantic Complexity   Semantic aspects of the stimulus (meaningfulness) have previously been noted to affect comprehension and production. The speed and accuracy of comprehension have also been found to increase and decrease, respectively, with increases in grammatical complexity (Baker and Holland, 1971; Lasky, Weidner, and Johnson, 1976; Levy and Holland; Shewan and Canter, 1971). This observation is well documented clinically by measures, such as the Token Test, which typically reveal increasing numbers of errors with increasing syntactic complexity.

Stimulus Presentation   The way the stimulus is presented has an effect on its ability to be recognized and produced. Weidner and Lasky (1976) investigated the effects of rate of presentation on auditory receptive performance of aphasic adults. Four auditory subtests of the Minnesota Test for the Differential Diagnosis of Aphasia were presented at 110 and 150 words per minute to aphasic subjects divided into two groups on the basis of Porch Index of Communicative Ability percentile scores. Results revealed that reducing the rate of presentation improved scores for each group and each task. A second study (Lasky et al., 1976) found that slower rate of presentation and the insertion of pauses at phrase boundaries had the effect of increasing correct performance. Moreover combining a slow rate and pauses, which allowed the greatest amount of auditory processing time, provided the highest number of correct responses for all levels of linguistic complexity studied, including active affirmative, active negative, and passive affirmative sentences. Similarly Liles and Brookshire (1975), utilizing the Token Test, found that the insertion of pauses generally had the effect of improving the ability to carry out commands.

Other aspects of stimulus presentation that improve performance include the number of modalities through which the stimulus is presented, the time during which the stimulus is available for processing, and the number of times the stimulus is presented. Multimodality sensory input of a stimulus, such as auditory and visual information simultaneously presented, has been demonstrated to improve naming compared to auditory or visual presentation alone (Gardiner and Brookshire, 1972). The positive effects of increasing the time during which the auditory stimulus is available for processing has an analogous situation in other modalities. Brookshire (1971b) found a gradual improvement in naming as the interval during which the visual stimulus was present increased under conditions of 3, 5, 10, and 30 seconds. The most successful condition in terms of number of correct responses per unit time occurred when the subject was allowed to determine how long the stimulus was available. Finally, it would be reasonable to expect that repeated presentations of auditory, visual, olfactory, or tactile stimuli would increase the probability of correct performance on the task.

The time between presentation of the stimulus and the patient's response —that is, the effect of imposed response delay—has also been studied. Yorkston, Marshall, and Butler (1977) investigated the effects of imposed response delay, the amount of sensory information available, and the interaction between these two variables. Utilizing a task similar to Part 1 of the Token Test, they presented commands auditorily only and then with auditory and visual information (subjects were allowed to see shapes during presentation and following the auditory stimulus) at response delays of zero, five, and ten seconds. Results revealed that the multisensory presentation group performed significantly better than did the auditory-alone group and that the imposed response delays had a positive effect on performance in the auditory plus visual presentation subjects. Yorkston et al. concluded that the response delay was not a limiting factor in the auditory-only group since it did not deteriorate their performance. For the auditory-visual group the response delay had the effect of providing extra processing time thereby improving performance and reducing the number of anticipatory errors.

Item Difficulty   Whether the patient is presented with a more or less difficult item quite obviously will affect performance. Additionally Brookshire (1972) has shown that ordering of easy and difficult items in series will affect naming. Utilizing a picture-naming task in which easy-to-name pictures were alternated with difficult-to-name pictures, he found that difficult items interfered with subjects' ability to name subsequent easy items, and conversely, easy items facilitated performance on subsequent difficult items. The ordering of stimuli, therefore, must be considered in the matrix of variables that determine the hierarchical difficulty of an item or task.

Context   The context within which the stimulus is presented may increase the likelihood of a correct response. Barton, Maruzewski, and Urrea (1969), using 48 aphasic subjects, evaluated the effects of three conditions on naming nouns: in response to pictures, within a clozentropy task ('To tell time we usually wear a———.''), and following a verbal description. They found that responses on the clozentropy task were least frequently in error, followed by naming in response to pictures and then verbal description. Similarly Hardison, Marquardt, and Peterson (1977) found that apractic subjects provided significantly more correct responses when the omitted noun in a clozentropy paradigm occurred toward the end rather than at the beginning of a sentence. Green and Boller (1974) investigated the effect of the grammatical form of a question or a command on the ability of aphasic subjects to respond. They found that there was no significant difference in percentage of correct responses between directly worded, indirectly worded, or introductory sentence stimuli. However when the responses were examined for appropriateness, significantly more responses were judged adequate when the form of the sentence was direct or contained an introductory sentence than when it was indirectly worded. Additionally Marshall (1978) reported on Marshall and Thistlethwaite's (1977) finding that an alerting signal improved performance on the Token Test for aphasic subjects.

Other factors having an impact on the potency of the stimulus or stimulus situation are the attitude of the clinician, prosodic aspects of the stimulus, and articulatory difficulty. Earlier it was noted that Stoicheff (1964) found that aphasic patients performed more poorly and rated their performance as poorer when presented with tasks with discouraging instructions compared to tasks with encouraging instructions. She proposed that discouraging instructions had the effect of increasing anxiety and reducing performance on the naming and reading tasks.

Stress appears to be influential in affecting task performance, especially for longer sequences. Goodglass (1973) observed that

> . . . production is facilitated by primary stress regardless of the grammatical function of the word tested; that is, stress factors neutralize the difference in production of grammatical and lexical items. Moreover, certain stress patterns override grammatical complexity. As a result, negative interrogative sentences are easier for aphasics to produce than simple interrogative sentences. These results suggest that linguistic impairment in aphasia cannot be explained exclusively by linguistic theories of derivational or transformational complexity but must be embedded in a performance model which considers other variables contributing to both production and comprehension. (p. 184)

Stress and perhaps other suprasegmental factors, therefore, interact with linguistic variables, and that interaction must be considered in predicting order of difficulty.

Phonetic (articulatory) factors affect the aphasic patient's verbal expressive skills. Most of the available data has been acquired from studies of apractic or Broca's aphasic patients. In general these studies (e.g., Hardison et al., 1977; Johns and Darley, 1970; Marquardt, Rinehart, and Peterson, 1979; Martin and Rigrodsky, 1974; Shankweiler and Harris, 1966) have found that fricatives, affricates, and consonant blends are most often misarticulated; vowels are more frequently produced correctly than are consonants; errors occur more frequently on nonmeaningful than on meaningful stimuli; errors increase with increases in word length above five phones; articulatory accuracy is affected by the frequency of occurrence of the phoneme; and errors are positively correlated with markedness and articulatory effort. Although these findings relate primarily to Broca's aphasics, Blumstein (1973) found similar distributions of errors (substitutions, simplifications, additions, contextual errors) and more substitutions from marked to unmarked than from unmarked to marked for three aphasic groups (Broca's, conduction, Wernicke's) which suggests a more universal effect for articulatory variables on the speech production accuracy of aphasic patients.

It appears, then, that almost every aspect of the stimulus situation impacts on the probability of obtaining a correct response from the patient and must be used in determining a difficulty hierarchy (see Table 4–2). Included are syntactic, semantic, phonological, and prosodic aspects of the stimulus; the attitude of the clinician; the time between the presentation of the stimulus and the patient's allowed response (imposed response delay); the number of modalities through which the stimulus is presented; the time during which the stimulus is available for processing; the intensity of the stimulus; and the ordering of easy and difficult items.

This, however, does not exhaust the variables in the stimulus situation that may affect performance. Bollinger and Stout (1976) noted that the number of choices in the response field from which the patient is to select the appropriate item affects the probability of a correct response. Although it is apparent that more choices in the field will produce more response errors, it is equally important to note that the characteristics of the response field choices will also have an effect; semantically and/or phonetically similar choices will produce a more difficult task (e.g., Rinnert and Whitaker, 1973).

○ CUES AND PROMPTS

Various cues and prompts may be presented to increase the likelihood of response accuracy (Table 4–2). These cues and prompts may be provided by the clinician or generated by the patient. Clinician-provided prompts are used to increase the potency of the stimulus so that it is sufficient to initiate an adequate response from the patient. The breadth of cues or prompts is large. McDearmon and Potter (1975) dichotomized those available. Association prompts were described as contextual cues which made the correct response highly predictable, such as, "We eat from a plate, we drink from a————." This is the sentence completion stimulus situation previously considered. Representational prompts, divided into two types, were described as stimuli which represented the concepts encompassed within the expected response. *Symbolic prompts,* according to McDearmon and Potter, are written, printed, or spoken words, whereas *realistic prompts*

TABLE 4-2

Stimulus Attributes, Prompts and Cues, and Facilitative Strategies

A. Characteristics of the clinician-controlled stimulus
  1. *Magnitude:*
    a. *Multimodality:* Presentation of a stimulus through more than one modality increases the liklihood of a correct response.
    b. *Size:* Larger visually presented items positively effect performance.
    c. *Ambiguity:* Whether presented auditorily or visually, less ambiguous stimuli enhance performance.
    d. *Intensity/competing noise:* Auditory stimuli presented at a moderate intensity without background noise are best.
    e. *Live voice:* Live voice presentation may be advantageous due to directly observable visual cues from the clinician.
    f. *Meaningfulness:* High frequency words of low abstraction level are most effective.
    g. *Length:* Shorter items, whether words or sentences, improve comprehension and production accuracy.
    h. *Operativity:* Use of items, or pictures of items, that can be manipulated improves performance.
    i. *Redundancy:* Repeated presentation or use of multiple cues increases frequency of correct performance.
  2. *Grammatical complexity:* Reduced grammatical complexity improves performance.
  3. *Stimulus presentation rate:* Performance is improved by reduced presentation rate, increased time of stimulus exposure, and imposed response delay.
  4. *Item difficulty:* Easy items improve performance on more difficult items that follow.
  5. *Context:* Use of multiple cues, introductory sentences, alerting signals and sentence completion tasks aid performance.
  6. *Stress:* Primary stress enhances word production regardless of grammatical function.
  7. *Articulatory factors:* Fricatives, affricates, and consonant blends are more difficult than other single consonants. Articulatory accuracy is affected by phoneme frequency of occurrence, markedness, and articulatory effort.
  8. *Clinician attitude:* Discouraging instructions may cause the patient to perform more poorly and to rate his performance as less satisfactory.
  9. *Response field number:* Less response field choices increases the liklihood of a correct response.

B. Cues and prompts: clinician provided or generated by patient.
  1. *Associational:* Stimuli containing contextual cues which make the response highly predictable. Included are the use of sentence completion, first sounds of words, superordinates, location, rhyme, and function.
  2. *Representational:* Stimuli representing the concept of the expected response.
    a. *Symbolic:* Written, printed, and spoken words.
    b. *Realistic:* Attributes of the stimulus such as a picture of the object, the object, or sensory properties of the object.

C. Patient-generated facilitation strategies: Activities the patient undertakes to trigger a correct response.
  1. *Delay:* Extra processing time is used or requested by the patient.
  2. *Association:* Words that are related to the target word are produced such as opposites, rhymes, and synonyms.
  3. *Description:* Characteristics of the concept are described such as size, shape, or function.
  4. *Generalization:* Use of general nonspecific terms.
  5. *Motor activity:* Gestures and tapping to improve speech production.

are attributes of the stimulus, such as a picture of the object, the object itself, or sensory properties of the stimulus, such as the smell of bread. The methodology in terms of using representational prompts, whether symbolic or realistic, is to yoke presentations of stimuli to elicit a response and then to gradually fade the prompts so that the patient can name, read, write, gesture, or perform whatever the expected response is with only a single representation of the stimulus present. For example, suppose an aphasic patient is asked to name a picture of a nurse, but the presence of the picture alone is not sufficient to evoke a correct response. However when a picture is accompanied by a nurse in the room (realistic prompt) and by silent oral production of the word by the clinician (symbolic prompt), the patient can say "nurse." Next, following repeated correct productions of the word, the stimulus situation is changed so that the clinician articulates the first sound of nurse and the patient continues to respond correctly. By gradual elimination (fading) of the symbolic (articulatory positions) and realistic (nurse) prompts, the patient reaches a point at which he or she correctly produces the word with only the picture of a nurse. This example assumes that both prompts are necessary to initially obtain successful performance of the task.

Pease and Goodglass (1978) examined the effects of six types of associative cues on naming. Twenty-four aphasic subjects were presented with pictures of objects; on those they failed to name correctly, cues were presented, and attempts at additional naming were recorded. First sounds, superordinates, location, rhyme, function, and completion were the cues used. A significant correlation was found between responsiveness to cuing and severity of aphasia. Whether divided by aphasia type or severity, first sound cues were most effective, followed by completion. Differential effects of superordinate, function, location, and rhyme cues were not significant.

Patient-generated cues are the activities the patient undertakes to facilitate a response. Berman and Peele (1967) noted that many aphasics have difficulty due to *associative interference*—that is, the production of a response that has an overt relationship to the correct response, such as a gesture, definition, or synonym. They observed that these associated responses sometimes trigger a correct response and reasoned that they might be used effectively to improve communicative performance. In five case reports of patients selected on the basis of their responsiveness to cues provided by the clinician, they reported the successful use of self-generated cues such as gestures, synonyms, opposites, rhymes, and reading aloud the initial sound of a word that produced correct production for the patients.

In a later study Marshall (1975) attempted ". . . (1) to identify the types of word retrieval strategies employed by aphasic adults in conversation, and (2) ascertain the relationship of these strategies to the 'triggering' of appropriate responses in conversation" (p. 166). Word retrieval problems of six aphasics in conversation were recorded, a determination was made as to whether the retrieval was successful, and the types of strategies used were noted. Four types of strategies were identified:

1. *Delay.* Extra processing time is used or requested by the patient.
2. *Association.* Words that are semantically related to the target word to be retrieved are produced, such as opposites, rhymes, and synonyms.
3. *Description.* Important elements of the concept to be retrieved are produced, such as those related to size, shape, or function.
4. *Generalization.* General nonspecific terms are used as a vehicle for retrieving the target word.

Marshall found that association and description were the most frequently used strategies, but that they were successful only approximately 50 percent of the time. Delay and generalization were used least often, with delay producing the most success and generalization the least. Also he noted that word retrieval strategies and aphasia severity appeared to be related—least involved patients were the only ones to use the most successful delay strategy and were generally more successful regardless of the word retrieval method used.

In a related study Farmer (1977) compared self-correctional strategies used by aphasic and nonaphasic brain-damaged subjects in conversation. Strategies were the same as defined by Marshall with the exception of the addition of a category entitled *sound revisions.* Although the total number of words produced by the two groups was not significantly different, the aphasic subjects used significantly more attempts at self-correction. When word retrieval frequencies were considered, delay was found to account for more self-correction occurrences than all other types combined. Additionally aphasics more often used description and generalization, and nonaphasics more often used association. Nonaphasics were more frequently successful at self-correction compared to the aphasic subjects. For both groups delay was most successful for self-correction, followed by association. Least success was produced by generalization. In a second part to the study Farmer found no significant differences in the percentage of successful self-correction as a function of type of aphasia although a significant correlation between success frequency and severity level was noted.

Several important statements may be drawn from this discussion of retrieval–self-correction–prompt–cuing strategies. First, aphasic patients spontaneously use strategies to aid in word retrieval. Second, clinician-generated cues add potency to the stimulus situation and increase the likelihood of a correct response. Third, self-generated cues can be effectively learned by the patient to enhance communicative effectiveness. If the use of self-generated cues is to be part of the therapy regime, LaPointe (1978) has outlined the steps to follow:

1. Identify and isolate effective cues.
2. Determine the skills necessary to the patient's volitional use of the cues.

3. Heighten the patient's awareness of the utility of the chosen cue for affecting correct responses.

4. Condition the patient to use self-produced cues. This may involve direct instruction of the strategy, indirect prompting and reinforcement. (p. 140)

Two additional issues—intersystemic reorganization and transcoding—need to be considered as part of this discussion. It has generally been observed that motor activity in the form of tapping (e.g., Sparks, Helm, and Albert, 1974) and gestures (Skelly, Schinsky, Smith, and Fust, 1974) have the effect of improving verbal expression. Intersystemic reorganization, attributed to Luria (1970), was defined by Rosenbek, et al. (1978), as ". . . the rebuilding of speech by the introduction into the act of speaking a system or set of responses in a unique form or with a unique regularity" (p. 315). Rosenbek et al. hypothesized that speech production is improved because associated gestures facilitate production and because gestures serve as a means of "speech reorganization." Consequently if manual gesturing and/or visual input (primary intersystemic reorganizers) are paired with auditory or tactile information and speech (oral gestures), it is suggested that speech production has been reorganized into a different functional system. One critical aspect of this process is that the reorganizer, such as manual gestures, must be intact in order to provide the basis for the reorganization. The primary reorganizer investigated to date is manual gestures paired with speech production, and the results have been mixed (Rosenbek et. al., 1978).

Related to intersystemic reorganization is the concept of deblocking the transcoding process. Transcoding was defined by Weigl (1974) as the ". . . relating of certain units in one sign system to corresponding units of another system" (p. 239). An example of transcoding would be writing to dictation where perceived auditory units are transcoded into graphic units. Weigl proposed that one effect of brain damage was to produce transcoding disorders which could at least be temporarily remedied by deblocking. Deblocking was described by Kreindler and Fradis (1968) as ". . . the possibility of obtaining for some time recovery of partially or totally lost language functions when the blocked performance is preceded by an appropriate nonblocked performance, provided both refer to the same word" (p. 150). For example, a patient has difficulty writing to dictation but not reading aloud. He is first presented the word to read aloud. Next, the target word is presented auditorily with others with the expected result that it will be written correctly. If a correct response is not obtained, the procedure is repeated. Kreindler and Fradis pointed out that the effect of deblocking is usually temporary (less than ten minutes) and that the effectiveness of the procedure is dependent on the integrity of the function used to produce the deblocking. It should be apparent that intersystemic reorganization and deblocking entail combining of intact and disordered functions in order to facilitate and reorganize speech and language processes, issues which have taken up much of the discussion to this point.

The review of stimulation and facilitation identified the variables to be considered in the construction of task hierarchies, but did not explore how they are to be selected for use in treatment. This topic will be covered in the discussion of specific therapy methods to follow and also later in the text. However, two points need to be made here. First, the variables cannot be assumed to be equally effective for patients with different neurogenic disorders or even for patients with the same diagnosis, Their effectiveness needs to be evaluated for each patient. Second, the possible combinations of variables is very large. It is not possible to systematically study all their additive and/or interactive effects for the next patient seen for treatment. The typical procedure is to utilize test results and informal assessment to identify those that are most helpful, and then to systematically explore various combinations to find the point at which the patient is partially, but not completely, successful to begin therapy.

○ SPECIFIC TREATMENT APPROACHES

Given the stimulation and programmed instruction rationales to treatment, the procedures attendant to these approaches, and the variables for constructing a stimulus hierarchy, specific treatment methods for neurogenic disorders can now be covered. The discussion will first consider two approaches combining features of stimulation and programmed instruction —Response Contingent Small-Step Treatment and Base-10 Programmed Instruction. Then methods directed at improving particular types of disorders such as apraxia and auditory comprehension deficits will be discussed.

response contingent small-step treatment (RCSST)

Bollinger and Stout (1976) described the RCSST as a structured behavioral methodology which

> ... enables the clinician to program treatment in such a manner that the patient proceeds from clinician-provided maximum external structure to maximum internal structure wherein the patient integrates and employs treatment strategies. Within such a treatment paradigm, the speech clinician provides external structure via a sequence of carefully controlled antecedent events and also acts as a feedback mechanism. This allows the communication disordered patient to work from highly structured specific response behaviors to more nondirected general language communication performances. (p. 41)

Basically the approach is similar to programmed instruction with the exception that greater attention is paid to the antecedent event than to the reinforcement of the response, and generalization of learned behaviors is anticipated. Implementation of the program requires determination of task hierarchies. Target behaviors are assumed to have a number of specifiable steps. The hierarchies reflect progression of the patient from heavily cued antecedent events with a small response field to low cued stimulus events and a large response field. Movement upward in the hierarchy then would reflect a successful response under conditions of less stimulus power and increased response field choices. Also to be determined are the response criterion and response constancy of the target hierarchy. *Response criterion* was defined by Bollinger and Stout as "... that level of performance established as a necessary prerequisite for successful performance of the next higher task" (p. 43) and *response constancy* as "... the number of items successfully completed at the required level of performance on that given task" (p. 44).

The program implementation for the patient initially involves presentation of the stimuli at maximum power—that is, with the most highly cued antecedent and a minimum number of choices in the response field. Single items are presented with decreasing power until the patient is unsuccessful. At this point the stimuli are presented at the preceding step in the hierarchy and multiple items presented until criterion level is reached. According to Bollinger and Stout, if the patient is not successful on four first-item presentations, the stimulus power–response field effects are not sufficient for eliciting successful performance, and the clinician should drop back to the preceding step and present items until the criterion level is reached. The next higher step can then be presented.

Two other important points are pertinent to this program. First, if there is a marked discrepancy between two steps, the program should be examined to determine whether an intervening step has been inadvertently omitted. If a step cannot be identified and the patient cannot reach criterion on the higher task, it is assumed the patient has arrived at a plateau in his or her progress. Secondly, a five-minute probe period is used at the beginning of each treatment session during which the patient is presented with stimuli above his or her current level of functioning. If the patient is successful at one of these higher levels, the intervening steps are omitted. This allows for skipping steps in the program during the course of language recovery.

A treatment record is produced in Figure 4–1. Included are spaces for indicating target behavior, input modality, output modality, stimulus, response criterion, and contingency. Following establishment of the patient's level of functioning via probing, the target behavior (T) and the next highest ($T + 1$) and next lowest ($T - 1$) steps of a given hierarchy are entered on the form. Three columns are provided so that data, as shown, can be recorded from three complete task presentations in terms of the stimulus presented, the response, and the contingency. Three types of contingencies

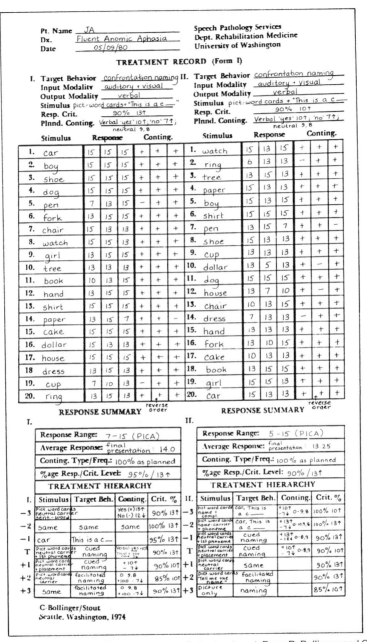

FIGURE 4–1 Treatment record for response small step treatment. From R. Bollinger and C. Stout, Response-contingent small-step treatment: performance-based communication intervention. *J. Speech Hearing* Dis., 41, 40–51 (1976). Reprinted by permission.

are used: positive, negative, and neutral. Presentation of a stimulus with successful response is followed with a positive contingency and an unsuccessful response by a negative contingency. If a response is not successful, the power of the stimulus is increased and/or the response field choices are decreased. When a successful response is obtained, a neutral contingency, such as "That's what you wanted," is provided. This, then, is the treatment. The patient is working at a level with a high frequency of success, yet one which is maximally taxing of his or her linguistic abilities. It should be noted that only the first response to an item is scored. Following an unsuccessful response, subsequent presentations of a stimulus at steps with more information provided are not recorded. The next scoring occurs with the presentation of the next stimulus item at the target level (T). The form also contains response summaries for planning future treatment sessions. Included are the response range, average response, contingency type/frequency, and percent responses/criterion level. A sample hierarchy containing 30 steps for a patient is provided in Table 4-3 from Bollinger and Stout. It should be noted, however, that the patient may not be required to complete each step in the program since recovery may negate the need for some levels of the treatment paradigm.

Several other points are relevant to this program. First, the program will typically include approximately 20 task items at each step. Secondly, Porch Index of Communicative Ability scoring is used, although other scoring systems may also be appropriate. Finally, the program is applicable to various types of disorders, such as aphasia, apraxia, and dysarthria, since the hierarchical system of stimulus difficulty would be necessary for treatment of each of these disorders.

Bollinger and Stout indicated that the RCSST allows for

> 1. Obtaining an accurate baseline of patient performance on a treatment-by-treatment basis which is often used to convey communication status to other staff members and third party providers;
>
> 2. Determining future small-step targets;
>
> 3. Increasing clinician observation of patient performance;
>
> 4. Enforcing more systematic treatment that is appropriate to the patient's level of ability;
>
> 5. Retrieving of information regarding language recovery patterns;
>
> 6. Providing for baseline behavioral determination when standard testing cannot be completed. (pp. 48–49)

RCSST is basically a programmed instruction approach to treatment which takes into consideration some of the principles of stimulation therapy previously described. Of particular interest is its detailed consideration of the many stimulus attributes that affect the potency of the antecedent.

TABLE 4–3

Sample Hierarchy for RCSST

The target behavior is an auditory-visual match in which the patient points to pictures named by the clinician. The input modalities are auditory and visual. The output modality is gestural.

	ANTECEDENT EVENT		RESPONSE CRITERION
	Power	*Number*	
1. Visual:	Corresponding picture and word.	Response Field: Two picture-word cards each presentation; One each monosyllabic and bisyllabic. One card repeated in each successive presentation over 20 trials.	100% of the responses should be at level of 10. Self-correct, or above; PICA scoring system.
Auditory:	Name said twice.		
Other:	High-frequency noun words, single and bisyllabic words equally represented.		
2. Same as 1.		Same as 1.	90% of the responses at level of correct or correct with delays; PICA scores 13 and above.
3. Same as 1.		Response Field: Two picture-word cards each presentation; One each monosyllabic and bisyllabic. One card repeated in each successive presentation over 20 trials.	90% of the responses should be at level of 10. Self-correct, or above; PICA scoring system.

Steps 4–16 are manipulations of single variables from power, number, or response criterion.

17. Visual:	Corresponding picture and word.	Response Field: Two picture-word cards each presentation. On each of 20 trials present two pictures not used on previous trials.	90% of the responses should be at level of 10. Self-correct, or above; PICA scoring system.
Auditory:	Name said once.		
Other:	High-frequency noun words, random monosyllabic presentation.		

Steps 18–29 are manipulations of single variables from power, number, or response criterion.

30. Visual:	Picture only.	Response Field: Eight picture cards each presentation. No cards from previous trials repeated in subsequent trials.	90% of the responses at the level of correct or correct with delay; PICA scores of 13 or above.
Auditory:	Name said once.		
Other:	High-frequency noun words, random monosyllabic presentation.		

From Bollinger, R., and Stout, C. Response-contingent small-step treatment: Performance-based communication intervention. *J. of Speech Hearing Dis.*, 1976, *41*, 40–51.

base-10 programmed stimulation

Base-10 Programmed Stimulation (LaPointe, 1977) is premised on a time series or subject as his or her own control design. Time series designs typically involve the establishment of a baseline (*A*) and measurement of behavioral change with institution of experimental procedures (*B*) to reveal the direction and magnitude of change. The design may be extended by discontinuing treatment to demonstrate, by return to baseline or plateauing of change, that behavioral alterations were a result of the experimental procedure and, further, by reinstating the procedures so that the final elaboration is repeated determinations of baseline and change as a consequence of implementation of the experimental or therapeutic procedures (A–B–A –B, and so on). A modification of this design, LaPointe noted, is suggested when a reversal of responses is unexpected or undesirable, as in language therapy. The modification is a multiple element or multiple baseline design which entails determination of baselines across behaviors, modalities, or patients. For example, baseline measurement of object recognition through tactile and visual modalities might be secured and therapy focused on visual object recognition. It is possible, however, to measure behavioral change through both modalities as a function of treatment focused in only the visual one.

Base-10 contains features of both programmed instruction and stimulation. Operant procedures include the measurement of baseline behavior, clear specification of tasks, and monitoring of change with institution of the therapeutic procedures. Stimulation therapy contributes concepts related to the sufficiency of the stimulus presented, the use of cues and prompts, and the need for continual and successful responses from the patient.

Examples of the Base-10 Response Form are presented in Figures 4–2 and 4–3. The form has space for indicating the task, defining and listing the criterion level, identifying the stimulus items used in the task, and for scoring performance on each item during each session. Ten items are selected, administered, and scored over ten therapy sessions. Correct or criterion performance is graphed to provide a pictorial display of progress.

The program does not specify what is to be worked on, nor does it indicate what contingencies are to be used. These decisions are end products of the evaluation and therapy planning. Rather, the program helps to organize the stimuli to be presented and to determine progress over repeated therapy sessions. The criterion level, stimulus items, and scoring system used are to be specified as part of the Base-10 program. The criterion level is not absolute and may vary, for example, from 80 percent acceptable performance over three trials on the stimuli chosen to 100 percent correct performance over more or less than three sessions. The stimulus items should be appropriate to the patient but, as noted earlier, are not dictated by the program except that there should be ten. The scoring system may be dichotomous (right or wrong); a multidimensional system, such as the Porch Index of Communicative Ability format; or some other qualitative system. If PICA scoring is used, the mean performance on the ten items is divided by 15 to determine a percentage for each session. Examples of PICA and dichotomous scoring on the Base-10 Response Form are provided in Figures 4–2 and 4–3.

Space is provided on the form for indicating baseline performance over three trials which may be obtained in one day or over several days. A requirement is that the baseline be stable so that departures with treatment

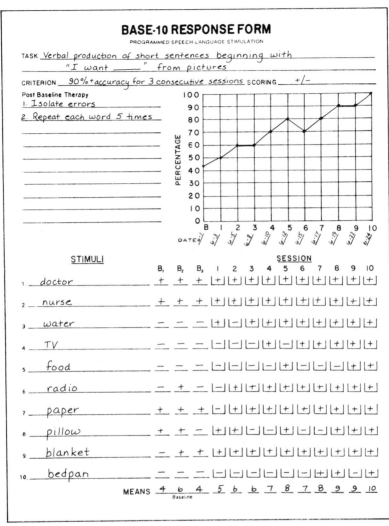

FIGURE 4–2 Sample Base-10 clinical treatment records showing plus-minus and Porch Index of Communicative Ability scoring. From L. LaPointe, *Base-10 Response Form.* Tigard, Oregon: C. C. Publications, Inc., (1979). Reproduced by permission.

can be reliably determined. Once baseline performance is determined, therapy is implemented. It is particularly noteworthy, and this point bears repeating, that Base-10 does not specify what the therapeutic procedures are to be. This is entirely the decision of the clinician. The type of treatment decided upon is specified by the clinician, however, on the form under the heading of postbaseline therapy. Performance during each session is re-tested and plotted over ten sessions if criterion is not reached before this point in the therapy regime.

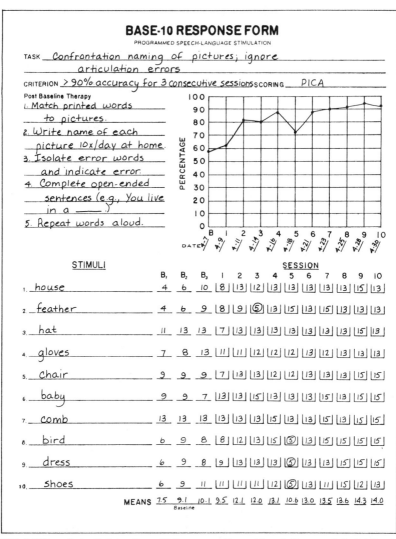

FIGURE 4-3 From L. La Pointe, *Base-10 Response Form*. Tigard, Oregon: C.C. Publications, Inc., (1979). Reproduced by permission.

clinician-controlled auditory stimulation for aphasic adults

Clinician-Controlled Auditory Stimulation for Aphasic Adults (Marshall, 1978) is a specific auditory approach to treatment with similarities to RCSST and Base-10. Marshall noted that from several recent studies (Czvik, 1976; Holland and Sonderman, 1973; Kushner and Winitz, 1977; West, 1973) "It is again becoming evident that auditory stimulation constitutes the foundation of aphasia treatment" (p. 2). The approach involves the presentation of a verbal message, which may be supplemented by visual and gestural input, to elicit a nonverbal response. Although the stimulus may be presented by tape recorder or live voice, Marshall emphasized that the clinician, rather than the program, is of critical importance. The verbal stimuli presented must be appropriate to the patient so that they "stimulate disrupted auditory processes" (p. 2). How the stimuli are to be presented to a particular patient is determined by analysis of the patient's responsiveness in light of situational, psychological, and physiological factors. Message delivery methods and stimulus attributes that have been demonstrated to improve the likelihood of a correct response were reviewed earlier. As part of that discussion, it was noted that the relative effects of each of the factors for a particular patient cannot be predicted. Consequently it is necessary for the clinician to systematically determine and document which combinations of techniques are maximally effective at producing a correct response. Message delivery techniques considered in Controlled Auditory Stimulation include rate of speaking, pause insertion, alerting signals, interstimulus pause time, response time, imposed response delay, stress, length of the stimulus presented, and semantic field (semantic or phonetic similarity of items in the response field).

Materials used in the program are 360 cards with pictured nouns divided into 60-pair sets which can be presented two, four, or six at a time. The cards are grouped so that syllabic length, the initial phoneme of the stimulus, and the number of semantically and phonetically related stimuli presented at one time can be controlled. To accomplish this control the three-card sets are each divided into five ten-pair groups. Group 1 nouns are monosyllabic and do not enjoy a close semantic or phonetic relationship. Group 2 items are based on the same criteria as Group 1 except they are polysyllabic. Group 3 nouns are semantically related between word pairs. Group 4 items are phonetically related between word pairs, and Group 5 nouns are semantically related within and between word pairs.

The recording form has three sections. Section One provides space for recording identifying information, noting factors that may affect performance, and describing the scoring system. Section Two is used to record the task, the stimulus presentation techniques used, the probe stimuli and responses, and 80 stimuli and responses from the treatment paradigm. Section Three is for summarizing patient performance, assessing results, and for planning future therapy. Notations of this section follow those of the Problem-Oriented Medical Record format which considers subjective and objective observations of behavior; assessment results to set the baseline, monitor progress, and determine prognosis; and short- and long-term therapy (treatment) plans.

Several systems for scoring responses may be used (e.g., plus-minus, PICA). However the recommended procedure is a multidimensional system derived from the PICA that considers the accuracy, responsiveness, and promptness of the response. Scores using this system range from 1 which is a "frank error, no response, rejection of the stimulus" to 8 which is an "accurate, responsive, prompt response."

As part of the treatment approach the task is described in detail, taking into consideration linguistic factors such as vocabulary and level of syntactic complexity, and a criterion level is established. The criterion level can be set as percent correct if a plus-minus system is used or by the percent of a given type of response obtained if multidimensional scoring is used.

A ten-item trial is used as a probe to determine which combinations of stimulus presentation techniques provide the most successful responses. For each probe the clinician must specify the techniques used and record the stimuli presented and responses obtained. Space for four probes are provided. Each probe serves as a determiner of how stimuli will be presented during the therapy session.

A completed Section Two of the response form (Figure 4–4) is included as an example. The task was identification of one of six semantically related nouns. The criterion was 80 percent or more of eight (accurate, responsive, prompt) or seven (accurate, responsive, minimally delayed) responses. Message delivery techniques for the first probe included reduced rate and insertion of a pause following the alerter "point to." There were six items in the response field, and the field was high (H) since stimuli were semantically related choices. Under these conditions the patient produced four responses of either seven or eight on Probe 1. The message delivery was altered for Probe 2 to include a delay between presentation of the stimulus and the patient's response which resulted in six responses of seven or eight. This presentation mode was then used for the task trials of ten items each. It can be seen that the patient reached criterion by Trial 4.

Marshall indicated that probes are to be used at the beginning of each session for each task to establish the message delivery technique. He also suggested that several tasks typically will be used in the same therapy session.

The stimulus cards provided can be manipulated in various ways. For example, they may be used for identification of nouns, function, noun and function, prepositions, affirmative and negative sentences, commands, and so forth.

melodic intonation therapy

Base-10 Programmed Stimulation and Response Contingent Small-Step Treatment provide forms into which are input stimuli based on the patient's demonstrated areas of communicative deficit. The framework for each approach allows the selection of content to be individually determined —there is no preset specification of candidacy or stimuli. To a more limited

SECTION TWO

Task Description: Identification of 1 of 6 semantically related nouns

Criterion: 80% or more 8 or 7 responses on two consecutive trials

Message Delivery Techniques

	Rate	Pause	Alerter	IPT	RT	Delay	Stress	Exposures	Field	Other
Probe 1	(–)	(✓)	"Point to"	( )	( )	( )	( )	(6)	H	
Probe 2	(–)	(✓)	"Point to"	( )	( )	(✓)	( )	(6)	H	
Probe 3	( )	( )		( )	( )	( )	( )	( )		
Probe 4	( )	( )		( )	( )	( )	( )	( )		

	Probe 1		Probe 2		Probe 3		Probe 4	
	Stimulus	Res.	Stimulus	Res.	Stimulus	Res.	Stimulus	Res.
1.	banana	6	apple	7				
2.	hospital	7	house	8				
3.	rain	2	snow	2				
4.	ear	7	nose	8				
5.	bed	8	chair	8				
6.	bee	2	spider	2				
7.	ambulance	3	boat	7				
8.	dime	8	penny	8				
9.	football	3	basketball	2				
10.	pants	2	tie	2				

Rate (+ faster, - slower); Alerter (indicate type); Pause, Interstimulus Pause Time, Response Time, Delay, and Stress (if used); Exposures (indicate number of choices in response field); Field (L if stimuli are phonetically and semantically unrelated, M if two or three related, H if four to six related); Other (indicate technique used).

FIGURE 4–4 Clinician controlled auditory stimulation for aphasic adults treatment record. Adapted from R. Marshall, *Clinical Controlled Auditory Stimulation for Aphasic Adults.* Tigard, Oregon: C. C. Publications, Inc., (1979). Reprinted by permission.

extent, due to the provision of stimulus materials, this is also true of Clinician-Controlled Auditory Stimulation. Melodic intonation therapy, on the other hand, provides structure for both content and form.

Melodic Intonation Therapy (MIT) has been reported to improve the expressive language abilities of severely impaired aphasic adults (Albert, Sparks, and Helm, 1973; Sparks et al., 1974; Sparks & Holland, 1976). The method focuses on the repetition of phrases in melodic intonation patterns which reflect the inflections, rhythm, and stress of normal speech. For patients who are successful with MIT, the results of treatment are impressive. Neurologically stable patients who have made minimal progress in therapy for several months with other approaches have progressed from no usable speech to the use of short, meaningful sentences within a relatively short period of time. However their speech remains agrammatic, and they do not improve significantly in auditory comprehension or reading, although their

TASK TRIALS

Trial 1

Stimulus: orange	church	sun	head	lamp
Response: 7	8	8	2	7
Stimulus: fly	plane	five dollars	bowling ball	hat
Response: 2	3	8	2	7

Trial 2

Stimulus: pear	theater	cloud	foot	table
Response: 8	3	7	8	7
Stimulus: bug	car	quarter	golf clubs	shirt
Response: 7	8	2	5	8

Trial 3

Stimulus: plum	school	stars	eye	rug
Response: 5	8	7	8	8
Stimulus: grasshopper	bus	nickel	tennis ball	gloves
Response: 2	8	8	7	8

Trial 4

Stimulus: lemon	barn	lightning	arm	desk
Response: 8	7	8	8	8
Stimulus: ant	train	one dollar	skis	coat
Response: 7	8	8	8	7

Trial 5

Stimulus:				
Response:				
Stimulus:				
Response:				

Trial 6

Stimulus:				
Response:				
Stimulus:				
Response:				

Trial 7

Stimulus:				
Response:				
Stimulus:				
Response:				

Trial 8

Stimulus:				
Response:				
Stimulus:				
Response:				

(Figure 4-4 continued)

response naming, confrontation naming, and phrase length are positively affected (Sparks et al., 1974).

Candidacy According to Sparks et al., the patients who benefit most from MIT include those who demonstrate auditory comprehension superior to verbal expression, reasonably intact attention span and emotional stability, severely restricted verbal output, and poor repetition skills. Helm (1976) investigated the correlation between patient variables and change in naming ability for a MIT-treated group of aphasics with relatively good auditory comprehension and severe verbal expression deficits. She found five variables which related to improved naming skills following MIT. Using these variables as predictors of success in MIT, she described the best candidates as those who begin therapy as soon as possible after onset of language impairment, demonstrate severe oral apraxia, use stereotyped syllabic jargon, and have poor word repetition skills. She minimized the significance of negative effects of surgery since the surgery in the patients studied was extensive. What might be concluded from these reports is that the primary candidates for the therapy are Broca's aphasics or mixed Broca's aphasics who demonstrate a severe apraxia of speech.

Procedures Few treatment approaches for aphasia consider as many variables relevant to successful rehabilitation of communicative functioning as does MIT. The treatment is hierarchically arranged into increasing levels of difficulty, baseline performance and criterion for successful performance is specified at each level, and stimuli are selected based upon phonological, semantic, syntactic, and suprasegmental factors.

Melodic Intonation Therapy uses a limited range of musical notes (three or four) which, according to Sparks and Holland (1976), approximate the range of inflection of American English. The application principle involved is that the prosodic pattern selected be appropriate to the inference intended for the sentence. The important elements of the intoned pattern are the melodic line, rhythm, and stress points. Under no circumstances are the intonation patterns of familiar songs used because they may generate regression to the words of the melody. Figure 4–5 shows three examples of melodic intonation patterns with the coding used to indicate melody, stress, and rhythm.

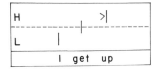

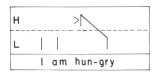

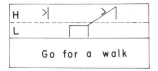

FIGURE 4–5: Melodic intonation patterns. | indicates single syllable word; ⊓ represents multisyllabic word or phrase; > indicates primary stress; *H* indicates higher than pitch; *L* represents lower than pitch.(Adapted from Sparks, R., and Holland, A. Method: Melodic intonation therapy for aphasia. *J. of Speech Hearing Dis.*, 1976, *41*, 287–297. Reprinted by permission.

Sparks and Holland (1976) noted that melodic intonation ". . . should have a slower and more lyrical tempo than speech, with more precise rhythm and more accentuated points of stress" (p. 289). They noted further,

> As the technique has developed, it has become clear that this divergence from speech facilitates articulation and reduces the frequency of paraphasic errors. Further, by directing the aphasic's attention to these three elements of melodic intonation—slow tempo, precise rhythm and distinct stress—the subject appears to be more capable of processing the structural aspect of the intoned verbal utterance (pp. 289–90).

MIT is divided into four progressive levels of difficulty with steps within levels. Level I has one step and involves the clinician humming a melodic pattern with a pitch range of three to four notes while aiding the patient in handtapping the rhythm and stress of the stimulus. This level is basically an orientation to the task. Level II, with five steps, progresses from nonverbal presentation of the stimulus by the clinician while assisting the patient in tapping on Step 1 to an intoned repetition of the stimulus by the patient in response to an intoned request by the clinician at Step 5. Level III, with four steps, introduces enforced response delays and requires the patient, at the final step of this level, to intone responses to intoned questions by the clinician regarding informational elements of the stimulus. Additionally, at Step 3 of this level, backups are introduced—that is, failure to perform correctly requires the patient to drop back one step in the program and to perform the sentence correctly before attempting the next higher level again. A second failure terminates work with that sentence. Backups are used whenever a stimulus above Step 3 of Level III is not produced correctly. Level IV is used to restore normal speech prosody. Longer phrases and longer imposed response delays are used with more complex phrases and sentences. Return to normal speech prosody is facilitated by the use of *Sprechgesang,* a technique which entails maintenance of the melodic line but replaces the constant pitch of intoned words with variable speech prosody.

The steps of the MIT program are hierarchically arranged in terms of difficulty so that, note Sparks and Holland, ". . . the aphasic patient is guided through a sequence of steps which increase the length of the units, diminish dependency on the clinician and diminish reliance on intonation" (p. 290). A gradual progression in the program is monitored by dichotomous scoring of the patient's responses on Levels II through IV. "Acceptable" performance is required at each step of these levels, and a 90 percent criterion based on the mean of ten consecutive scores (sessions) has been established for progression from one level to the next. Items may be repeated to improve scores if the patient's performance is not adequate at a level of the program.

Stimuli Stimuli are 12 to 20 phrases or sentences at each level. It is suggested that they be relevant to the patient's needs and background. Level II stimuli should not exceed four words, while longer and more complex sentences are used at Levels III and IV. At each level a patient progresses through the steps until the item is failed or successfully completed.

Additional definition of the stimuli to be used continues to evolve. Helm (1977) suggested that phonological and syntactical aspects of the stimuli be considered in the construction of the sentences. She indicated that the progression from easiest to most difficult phoneme classes was bilabials, alveolars, velars, sibilants, and affricates and that blends and words with an initial vowel were difficult to produce. She further noted that imperative sentences with initial intransitive verbs *(shut the door)* be used because they have facilitative first-syllable primary stress and allow the patient to effectively manipulate his or her environment. Sparks and Holland (1976) observed:

> It is clear that careful attention to the grammatical structure of language units is now in order, perhaps in terms of gradual increase of linguistic complexity, perhaps in terms of linguistic spontaneity by using a changing lexicon in appropriate slots of controlled and defined sentence types, or perhaps in some other as yet unspecified way. (p. 291)

Modifications of procedures and content for aphasic patients have been reported by Dunham and Newhoff (1979), Marshall and Holtzapple (1976), and Sparks (1981).

MIT is noteworthy for several reasons. First, the procedures to be applied are explicit and replicable with specific information provided on form and content. Second, it capitalizes on a large body of data relative to phonological, syntactic, semantic, and suprasegmental attributes of the stimulus and the positive effects of motor activity accompanying speech production. Finally, it has the semblance of a neurophysiological rationale (Berlin, 1976; Sparks, et al., 1974) to account for its success. It is hypothesized that MIT emphasizes the right hemisphere's use of the prosodic elements of speech which in turn enhances its role in the interhemispheric control of language via transcallosal pathways.

integral stimulation

Another treatment method developed specifically for apraxia is the eight-step continuum proposed by Rosenbek, Ahern, Harris, and Wertz (1973). It is similar to the other specific methods discussed in that there is a movement from maximum use of stimulus input with gradual reduction of the cues available until ultimately there is a transition to more typical communicative situations. The steps include:

Step 1. Patient is instructed to watch and listen carefully as the clinician models the utterance (integral stimulation) followed by simultaneous production of the utterance by clinician and patient.

Step 2. Integral stimulation followed by delayed production of the utterance with only visual cues (clinician mimes utterance as patient produces it aloud).

Step 3. Integral stimulation followed by delayed production of the utterance by the patient without visual and auditory cues.

Step 4. Integral stimulation followed by repeated production of the utterance by the patient without auditory or visual cues.

Step 5. Presentation of a written visual stimulus and simultaneous production of the utterance by clinician and patient.

Step 6. Production of the utterance by the patient after a written stimulus has been presented and removed.

Step 7. Utterance produced by patient in response to a question by the examiner.

Step 8. Appropriate use of the response during role playing.

To complete the brief review of specific methods that emphasize the rehabilitation of speech and language, two therapy approaches directed toward improving naming skills will be presented.

semantic, oppositional, rhyming, retrieval training (SORRT)

SORRT is a word retrieval program developed by Dixon and Logue (1980) for anomic patients. Use of the program is preceded by a series of probes to demarcate the patient's primary types of responses and retrieval behaviors and, importantly, to identify those that are seldom or ineffectually used. The 20-item probes include free association (to determine the incidence of between- versus within-noun class responses), semantic association (responses similar or identical in meaning to the stimulus), oppositional association (responses opposite in meaning to the stimulus), and rhyming association (responses which rhyme with the stimulus word). Additionally a 300-word conversational speech sample is obtained and analyzed according to the categories established by Marshall (1975). These categories, reviewed earlier, include delay, semantic and phonetic association, description, and generalization. This analysis yields the total number of errors, retrieval strategies used, and their effectiveness and accuracy in conversation. The probes are to be administered as a prelude to and over the course of treatment to determine progress. The word retrieval program is geared toward working on those retrieval skills (semantic, oppositional, rhyming) that are most impaired by means of a three-phase program for each retrieval area.

The first phase (auditory discrimination) requires the patient to make same-different judgments regarding word pairs presented auditorily. In the second phase (selection) the patient matches a visually presented stimulus to one of three words on the same card after reading the four-word list. The stimulus word and response chosen are then repeated. On the generative task (the third phase) the patient verbally responds to an auditorily presented word (cued visually and auditorily, if necessary). During each phase of the three retrieval task areas (semantic, oppositional, rhyming), feedback is provided by the clinician regarding the accuracy of the response. If a response is in error, the clinician explains to the patient why it is unacceptable. Criterion at each phase is 90 percent accuracy over two trials, and a record is to be maintained regarding the percentage of accuracy, type of error substitution, and degree of self-correction at each phase. When the third phase (generative) of a program area is completed, the assessment probes are readministered. Typically the weakest retrieval area is treated first. However all three areas may be treated at the same time with the major emphasis on the most impaired retrieval behavior.

Three across-class sorting tasks are also included: auditory-visual sorting (placing cards containing word pairs in categories identified as "opposites," "rhymes," or "means the same" after reading them aloud); auditory discrimination sorting (verbally stating whether word pairs presented auditorily best fit semantic, oppositional, or rhyming categories); and generative sorting (patient provides opposite, rhyming word, or synonym in response to auditorily presented word). Criteria for auditory-visual and auditory discrimination sorting has been set at 90 percent; for generative sorting, 80 percent.

Based on this description, it should be apparent that SORRT is appropriate for the mildly to moderately involved patient owing to the necessary reading and auditory comprehension skills for successful completion of the program. Next to be considered is a therapy intervention method that makes important distinctions in the types of naming behaviors to be treated.

divergent and convergent semantic therapy

Chapey (1977) found that aphasic patients are impaired in both convergent and divergent semantic behaviors—that is, they demonstrate difficulty in providing previously learned semantic information when a specific response is required (I eat from a plate, I drink from a———) and in generating a variety of relevant responses to a given topic (list all objects made of glass). She noted further (1981) that most therapy programs for aphasia are concerned with convergent behaviors—the patient is required to provide an agreed-upon response to a stimulus or to describe a specific picture, action, or event. Since convergent and divergent semantic behav-

iors are critical to language use, she proposed that therapy should emphasize both behaviors. Divergent therapy, according to Chapey, should first
emphasize orientation and attention by requiring the patient to observe, via
videotape, the divergent semantic behaviors used by normal speakers. During this phase all visual and auditory orientation behaviors of the patient are
reinforced. As divergent verbal responses are initiated in response to the
task, they too are immediately reinforced in order to increase their number
and variety. Additional tasks are described that have been found to stimulate
divergent semantic behaviors in normal speakers with the implication being
that they might effectively be used with aphasic patients.

Chapey (1981) described a sample divergent-convergent semantic
therapy program. Basically, it involves requesting divergent verbal responses (e.g., list all the things that burn) followed by convergent techniques such as description, copying, and identifying to increase the number
of responses. The convergent and divergent responses are then integrated
by requesting the patient to respond to a divergent task for which the newly
retrieved alternatives would be appropriate. Following each divergent task
the number and variety of responses are tabulated to monitor the effects of
treatment. For the convergent task, PICA scoring may be used and self-
cuing strategies taught to improve the retrieval behavior.

○ NONSPEECH COMMUNICATION TECHNIQUES

The foregoing discussion has emphasized the therapy forms and
content most frequently used to reestablish communication by verbal (audi-
tory-vocal) means. This is not to say that techniques such as Base-10 and
RCSST do not allow for the use of nonvocal therapy content but rather to
point out that the primary intent of most therapy strategies is to redevelop
typical premorbid verbal functioning.

Many neurogenic patients, because of motor or linguistic deficits, are not
able to use oral speech and must rely on nonvocal systems exclusively for
communication or at least must supplement their communicative efforts
with nonspeech modes. Silverman (1980) defined a nonspeech communication mode as ". . . any approach to encoding and transmitting messages that
does not require a person to *directly* produce speech sounds . . ." (p.3). He
defined three nonspeech modes—gestural, gestural-assisted, and neuro-
assisted. Gestural modes include gestures and movements through which
encoded messages are visually transmitted and include American Indian
sign language, gestural Morse code, pointing, and so forth. Gesture-assisted
modes are characterized by the use of movements or gestures which produce a display of the message to be conveyed. Examples are communication
boards, typewriters, speech synthesizers, and various symbol systems. Bio-
electrical signals are used to activate a readout device or display in neuro-
assisted modes.

Silverman noted that there are more than 100 systems for encoding and transmitting messages by nonspeech communication modes. The intent here is to provide examples of gestural and gestural-assisted modes that are frequently used with neurogenic patients. Neuro-assisted modes will not be considered not only because they are infrequently available for use by the communicatively handicapped patient with an acquired neurogenic disorder but also because they have several disadvantages. The disadvantages, according to Silverman, are that these modes tend to cost more, tend to transmit messages at a slower rate, are more likely to malfunction, must be attached to the user, and are not as highly developed as gestural or gestural-assisted modes.

gestural mode: American Indian Hand Talk (Amer-Ind)

Although a number of gestural communication systems have been developed for use with neurogenic patients (e.g., Chen, 1968, 1971; Eagleson, Vaughn, and Knudson, 1970), the adaption of American Indian hand talk by Skelly and associates (1974, 1975, 1979) has gained the widest acceptance and use. Skelly suggested that any gestural system for the speechless should be judged on the basis of six criteria. The system should

1. Have a low level of symbolism with a concrete reference base for the gestures.
2. Be easily acquired by the speechless patient.
3. Be readily interpreted by the speechless patient's audience.
4. Be flexible in the encoding of concepts.
5. Have a high degree of adaptability to existing gestures.
6. Have a potential speed of execution greater than that of written communication.

She concluded that Amer-Ind meets these requirements:

> The American Indian Code's low symbolic level, ease of acquisition, flexibility, speed, lack of grammatical structure and rules, and use of concrete, demonstrable referents, which enable the viewer to interpret without formal instruction, make it adaptable to the use of many patients unable to speak. It can also be of special value to those speechless patients who, through brain damage, are unable to use other gestural systems. (1979, p. 7)

Amer-Ind has approximately 250 clinically tested signals which allow the concepts of the 1,000 most-used English words to be expressed. Individual gestures may be used to express a concept, or gestural elements can be used in combination (agglutination) to convey a concept for which one signal is insufficient or does not exist.

Amer-Ind signals are action-oriented kinetic pictographs used to transmit concepts telegraphically. They are highly iconic, but a single gesture may convey a different meaning depending on the communicative context. For example, the gesture for *eat* may also be interpreted as *feed, food, hungry, meal,* or *nourish.* The signals are classified according to their manner of production: static, kinetic, or repetitive. Static signals consist of a single hand gesture held in position; kinetic gestures involve the use of a specific movement; repetitive signals transmit the concept by three repetitions of the movement. Only approximately 20 percent of the signals require the use of two hands so that the gestural code is particularly appropriate for the hemiplegic patient. The agglutinated gestures for conveying *cat* and *hospital* are shown in Figure 4–6. Gestural elements for *cat* are *animal* and *mustache;* for *hospital, shelter* and *pain.* Skelly provides more than 100 suggested agglutinations but many more are possible.

A scale of progress, divided into ten levels, has been developed for Amer-Ind. The first four levels are termed *preuse* and include stimulation for minimal response and signal recognition, execution, and retrieval. The fifth level is termed *transitional* and involves the use of signals with appropriate persons within the clinic (e.g., staff members, other patients, visitors) and other environments (e.g., home, stores, church). The next three levels are termed *signal use* and include self-initiated gestures, spontaneous conversation, and gestural use equivalent to propositional speech. The final two levels are *transfer stages* and involve the use of gesture to facilitate oral expression or as support for verbal expression.

The scale provides both a quantitative and qualitative estimate of the patient's level of functioning. A quantitative description is obtained by recording the number of signals available to the patient for communication and a qualitative description by the levels at which they are used. By noting the highest and lowest levels at which a signal or signals are used, a range of usage is obtained.

gesture-assisted modes

As described previously, gesture-assisted modes are communication systems that allow the message to be displayed, including typewriters, symbol systems, speech synthesizers, and so forth. One frequently used gesture-assisted communication device is the communication board (Figure 4–7). This rudimentary system allows the patient to indicate his or her primary needs by pointing, assuming that he or she is able to recognize the pictures and/or words provided. It is not intended to ensure a communica-

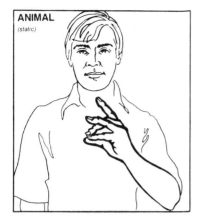

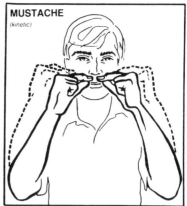

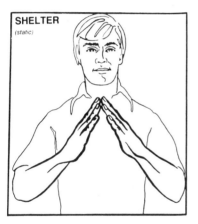

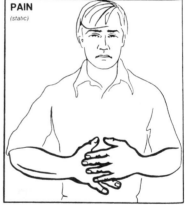

FIGURE 4–6 Agglutinated Amer-Ind signs depicting *cat* and *hospital*. Adapted from Skelly M. *Amer-Ind Gestural Code Based on Universal American Indian Hand Talk.* New York: Elsevier North Holland, 1979. Reprinted by permission.

tion device for the long term; more flexible and comprehensive systems should be developed as soon as possible.

Experimentation has also been directed toward the development of a gesturally assisted symbol-based system. Glass, Gazzaniga, and Premack (1973) studied seven patients with global aphasia. Using cutout paper symbols for words, they found that these patients were able to attain various levels of ability ranging from expression of same-different distinctions to simple action statements. They concluded that global aphasics retained at

INITIAL COMMUNICATION CHART FOR APHASICS

A NURSING HOME SERVICE PROGRAM PROVIDED BY MARION PHARMACEUTICAL DIVISION

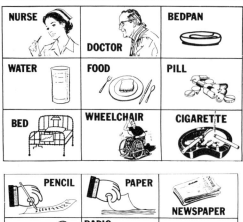

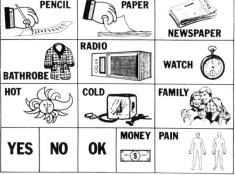

FIGURE 4–7 Initial Communication Chart for Aphasics. Courtesy of Marion Laboratories, Inc., Kansas City, Missouri.

least some symbolization and linguistic functioning in the presence of massive dominant hemisphere brain damage.

In a later study Gardner, Zurif, Berry, and Baker (1976) investigated the ability of severely involved global aphasic patients to use a symbol-based system. The system, termed *Visual Communication* (VIC), consisted of denotatively meaningful geometric and ideographic forms drawn on movable index cards, one symbol per card. The communicative interchange, which was nonverbal, involved the patient or clinician placing a series of cards in front of the other and the respondent selecting appropriate cards from his or her own set or carrying out an appropriate response.

Two levels of the system were identified. Level 1 was used to teach three functions: carrying out commands, answering questions, and describing events. If Level 1 was mastered by the patient, Level 2 was initiated, which entailed exploration of the ability to express needs and desires. Syntax using the symbols was linearly ordered with the agent appearing first, followed by the objects, locations, and beneficiaries of the action. The set for Level 1 was very restricted and consisted of five verbs, seven nouns, and three grammatical morphemes. The study was limited to five treated patients, all of whom completed Level 1 and two who completed both levels. Finding that the subjects' use of VIC was superior to their use of English, Gardner et al. concluded that the severely involved aphasics were capable of mastering an alternative symbol-based system. VIC is not a gesturally assisted communicative strategy currently in clinical use, but it has been instrumental in the development of Visual Action Therapy, a gesture-based treatment method.

Visual Action Therapy (VAT) for global aphasics was described by Helm and Benson (1978). It resembles VIC to the extent that the patient ". . . is trained to associate ideographic forms with particular objects and actions, and to carry out a series of tasks in association with these drawings" (p. 2). The assumption is that the understanding and production of symbolic gestures might serve as an early step in language treatment. Eight manipulable objects, such as a cup or razor, eight large and small line drawings of the objects, and eight pictures of the objects being manipulated serve as materials. The three-level program does not use verbalization. Level 1 uses objects and has 12 steps which progress from tracing the picture of the object at Step 1 to producing a representational gesture to symbolize an object no longer in view at Step 12. Levels 2 and 3 duplicate the last six steps of Level 1. However action cards and small picture cards, respectively, are substituted for the objects. Helm and Benson reported that seven global aphasic patients who had received VAT showed improvement based on Boston Diagnostic Aphasia Examination and Porch Index of Communicative Ability test scores on skills such as naming and writing, and particularly in auditory comprehension and gestures. Three of the patients were sufficiently improved to qualify for Melodic Intonation Therapy which, as noted earlier, requires relatively good auditory comprehension skills.

○ TREATMENT EMPHASIZING COMMUNICATIVE INTERACTION

The primary emphasis in the early part of this discussion was with the restablishment of the semantic/syntactic/phonologic/suprasegmental aspects of language for the neurogenic patient with considerably less attention paid to its use in everyday situations. The concern was with rationales, stimulus attributes, and therapy forms and content as they reflect the steps necessary for reacquisition of speech and language. The focus in this "traditional" approach is on verbal accuracy rather than communicative efficiency. For example, suppose *chair* is the focus of treatment. The task may be for the patient to produce the word. Depending on the severity of the patient's disorder, more or less information is provided to increase the saliency of the stimulus and thereby elicit a correct (verbally accurate) response. The stimulus may be presented through more than one modality (oral presentation of the word coupled to a picture of a chair), it may be presented repeatedly before a response is requested, and/or it may be presented within a sentence frame with or without an imposed time delay. The emphasis is on stimulus adequacy, stimulus-response drill, learning, and verbal accuracy to develop usable speech and language. This holds true whether the treatment is based primarily on programmed instruction (e.g., Response Contingent Small-Step Treatment) or stimulation (e.g., Clinician-Controlled Auditory Stimulation for Aphasics) rationales. Further it is clearly obvious that the purpose of approaches such as Melodic Intonation Therapy is to develop verbal production of phrases and/or sentences (*sit on the chair*) so that they will be available when a communicative situation is presented.

Concern has been expressed recently with the validity of standard appraisal instruments as indicants of communicative ability and with the underlying premises of treatment paradigms that stress verbal accuracy rather than communicative efficiency. The Functional Communication Profile and Communicative Abilities of Daily Life assessment instruments, for example, were developed because it was obvious that aphasia and related disorders may affect language processing to a greater extent than communicative competence. This is readily apparent in the clinical setting where patients communicate more effectively than their test scores on aphasia batteries would indicate. Their verbalizations may be circumlocutionary and heavily supplemented with gestures, but their communicative efforts are successful. The greater communicative integrity of patients with aphasia has also been documented in controlled experiments. For example, Wilcox, Davis, and Leonard (1978) found that aphasic patients demonstrated indirect-request contextual comprehension abilities that were superior to their performance on a standard comprehension battery. They concluded, "Standard tests of auditory comprehension . . . offer a measure of aphasic breakdown in linguistic processing but do not adequately reflect aphasics' receptive abilities in natural communicative settings" (p. 362).

The observation that communicative ability is more intact that language processing has led to a call for treatment approaches that capitalize on the residual abilities of the patient. In a discussion of the applications of speech acts (Searle, 1969) and language pragmatics (Ervin-Tripp, 1975) to aphasia treatment, Holland (1975, 1978) noted:

1. Contexts other than nonfunctional didactic settings must be utilized in treatment.

2. There should be increased concern with relevant (useful) language and communication. Helping the patient to communicate his or her needs is more important than the language structures used to convey the message. The language forms addressed in treatment should be decided upon by what is most necessary for the patient to communicate effectively in everyday situations.

3. It is necessary to observe and be sensitive to how aphasic patients communicate. In other words, an effort should be made to reinforce and enhance compensatory communicative behaviors of the patient.
4. Unconventional communicative strategies of the patient should be capitalized on.

In a discussion of treatment, Holland (1978) noted that two aspects of functional communication were relevant to aphasia rehabilitation and could be reduced to two questions: "What is a functional response?" and "What are functional stimuli?"

What constitutes a functional communicative response, according to Holland, involves consideration of three factors: (1) the strategies used by the patient to get the message across, (2) compromises on accuracy that are acceptable to the patient and his or her family, and (3) the use of alternative modes of communication. In other words, a functional response is a communicative behavior that effectively conveys an intended message, that can consistently be used by the patient even though it is not verbally accurate, and that may entail the use of other than a verbal mode, such as a communication board, or other gesture or gesture-assisted modes.

It is noteworthy that many patients spontaneously develop compensatory communicative strategies. For example, when an insurance salesman with aphasia and severe verbal apraxia secondary to a left cerebrovascular accident was asked where he worked, he first attempted to produce the name of the company verbally. Unable to do so after repeated trials, he tried to write it but could only write the first letter of the company's name. After a moment of thought, he took out his wallet and produced an insurance company identification card. The point to be made is that aphasic patients can be effective communicators even though language and verbal expression are severely impaired. According to Holland, the following therapy questions should be answered if functional responding is to be developed: Which of the patient's strategies should be capitalized on and reinforced? Which can be made more effective? When should alternative modes of communication be employed to develop functional responding?

The relevant aspects of functional stimuli, according to Holland, can be determined from the everyday communicative activities of the patient and the communicative acts that are encompassed in the performance of these activities. Communicative activities include such things as reading the mail and newspapers, writing notes and checks, looking up phone numbers and addresses, asking the location of items in a store, meeting a salesperson at the door—in other words, activities engaged in by the patient in a typical day. The communication acts involved with these activities include agreeing, denying, requesting, furnishing information, and so forth, many of which have gestural equivalents. Functional tasks in treatment, then, might include ordering a meal from a menu within a specified price range, balancing the checkbook using small and large numbers, requesting the location of grocery store items, and so on. These activities, as noted by Holland, can be hierarchically arranged in difficulty and are amenable to Base-10 recording.

promoting aphasics' communicative effectiveness

Closely allied to the functional treatment described by Holland is Promoting Aphasics' Communicative Effectiveness (PACE). Four principles underlie the procedures of PACE (Wilcox & Davis, 1978):

1. New information is conveyed by the clinician or patient—only one of the persons at the beginning of the communicative interchange has information regarding the message to be conveyed.
2. The patient may use any modality or combination of modalities to convey the new information. The clinician ensures that all communication modalities are available by means of modeling but does not direct the patient in terms of which ones to use.
3. The clinician and the patient are equal participants as senders and receivers of information.
4. Feedback is provided by the clinician in the form of acknowledgment that the message has been successfully conveyed or received.

An example of PACE therapy would be for the clinician and the patient to take turns communicating the names of objects depicted on cards with the clinician modeling available modalities such as gesturing, pointing, or verbally presenting the name of the object and the patient responding, followed by a reversal of the sender-receiver roles. A second functional method was developed by Cochran (1980).

conversational prompting

Cochran (1980) observed that most therapy programs for aphasia develop isolated, rather than comprehensive, communication skills—that is, they focus on language skills rather than the contexts in which they are used. Conversational prompting was developed to allow the patient to use appropriate responses rather than learned and habituated behaviors that might not be appropriate to the communicative context. Prompting is composed of a series of tasks graduated in difficulty, including communicative interaction related to object manipulation; performance of stories, events, and sequences with and without props; picture description; event description; structured questions and answers; structured and unstructured discussion; and free conversation. The topics include activities, such as taking a bath, going to dinner, or attending church, that are known to both the patient and clinician. The clinician initiates the conversation regarding the topic and provides whatever prompts are necessary for the patient to produce a response appropriate to the context. If the response cannot be understood, the clinician may guess or request additional information. What the patient does determines what the clinician does next. In other words, over repeated trials, whatever prompts are necessary for the patient to retrieve the response are provided. Included are situational context, clozenthropy, auditory and visual phonetic cues, intonational and stress prompts, paraphrasing, gesturing, modeling, and feedback. The prompts are then gradually reduced until the patient can produce the response without any aid from the clinician. A series of contextually useful responses are developed. Conversational prompting differs from traditional methods in that (1) the focus is on the two-way conversational turn-taking interaction between speaker and listener, (2) there is a continual effort on the part of the clinician to maximize the communicative success of the patient, and (3) the context is emphasized rather than specific stimulus drill.

Traditional and *functional* therapies are not necessarily at cross-purposes. Regardless of theoretical orientation, most clinicians would agree that the materials (stimuli) chosen for therapy should emphasize the concepts most necessary for the patient to communicate his or her needs and by doing so to control, at least in a limited way, the environment in which he or she resides. They would also agree that the goal of treatment is to maximize the communicative effectiveness of the patient. They clearly differ, however, in emphasis. Traditional approaches stress language structure and form. Functional therapy concentrates on intent, function, and use. It is obvious that some of the didactic procedures of traditional methods limit the variety of speech acts (Wilcox and Davis, 1977), but in many cases, their intent is to develop concepts necessary for communication but which are not available for use. Functional therapy, on the other hand, assumes that communication concepts are available but require the development of strategies for their effective use. Both approaches would appear to have a place in rehabilitation of the neurogenic patient—a topic to be covered in the next chapter on the rehabilitation process.

○ GROUP THERAPY

The confluence of therapy forms and content is in group treatment. Included within this approach are forms from programmed instruction (Holland, 1970) to academically based stimulation (Wepman, 1947); content from Melodic Intonation Therapy (Sparks et al., 1974) and Amer-Ind to psychiatric counseling (Blackman and Tureen, 1948); and disorder groups as diverse as multiple sclerosis (Long, 1954), Parkinson's disease

(Chafetz, Bernstein, Sharpe, and Schwab 1955), and aphasia, as well as their families (Redinger and Dolphin, 1970). The one common feature of group therapy programs is that one or more persons besides the patient and the clinician are active participants in the communicative situation. Although its lack of regimented procedures and its stated multiple purposes may initially appear to make it of less value than more goal-directed therapy forms, its record of longevity in the treatment of neurogenic patients suggests that it holds important advantages.

In a review of reports of group treatment approaches, Marquardt, Tonkovich, and DeVault (1975) cited the advantages attributable to group therapy:

1. Provides an opportunity for rehabilitative staff to study the patient and his or her needs, as well as a social setting in which the aphasic's interaction with others can be critically evaluated in terms of communicative content and facility.

2. Provides the patient with an opportunity to carry over newly developed communicative strategies into "real-life" situations. While somewhat artificial, such situations supply the patient with experiences beyond the one-to-one individual therapy sessions and afford him or her the opportunity to communicate before or within a group.

3. Provides psychological support in the form of sympathy, encouragement, humor, and understanding. In the group context, family members and patients can benefit from the experiences and emotional support of others in dealing effectively with their own situations.

4. Acts as an instrument of clinician training.

5. Exposes the patient to a variety of communicative strategies. The patient is able to observe the techniques used by other aphasic patients to communicate information.

6. Provides motivation, stimulation, and friendly competition. The group situation provides an opportunity for motivation from peers. It apparently is easier for the aphasic to attempt an appropriate response if another patient, who has failed initially, becomes successful on the second or third attempt.

7. Provides a social situation based on a common need for communication and language retraining. The aphasic patient is often not able to socialize easily with verbally unimpaired persons. Socialization is facilitated when the patient is incorporated into a group of similarly handicapped individuals.

8. Provides a setting in which conflict can be ventilated and acted out in a controlled manner.

9. Serves as an adjunct to individual speech and language retraining and results in more consistent language recovery.

Disadvantages of group treatment include:

1. May make it difficult for withdrawn patients to attempt expression.
2. May be paced too slowly for faster learners in a group and too fast for slower learners.
3. May provoke talk of personal problems before the patient is ready to make such revelations.

If the purposes of group treatment are examined, three primary goals are evident. First, it has served as a means of providing direct speech and language treatment when trained personnel were in short supply (such as during World War II) or of providing controlled communicative situations in which the patient could use newly developed strategies. Second, group therapy has been used for socialization within an informal setting where friendships and camaraderie can be developed. Third, group settings have served the purpose of dealing with the emotional reactions of the patient and family. It is important to point out that none of these purposes is independent, and goals are determined more by the professionals who lead the group than by the most immediate problems of the patients. For example, in a meeting of patients set up by a speech-language pathologist, the purpose will typically be to improve speech and language skills. However, to a limited extent at least, patients will socialize and discuss at least some of their emotional responses to their common bond—acquired brain damage. If a psychiatrist led the group, on the other hand, emotional issues might be the primary topic, but communicative activities and socialization would also occur.

This chapter was concerned with treatment forms and content. Rationales, stimuli, procedures, and the theoretical underpinnings and data-based support for approaches were emphasized. The focus was on the therapy methods available rather than on when and with whom particular procedures were to be employed. Also evident was the fact that little mention was made of treatment for neurogenic disorders besides aphasia and apraxia. These issues will be considered further in the following chapter which will address longitudinal aspects of rehabilitation for neurogenic communication disorders.

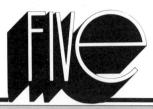

The rehabilitation process

○ INTRODUCTION

Evaluation, prognosis, and therapy are integral, overlápping components of rehabilitation. Discussion of these topics, however, did not yield a format for the process or information on the full range of activities involved. The purpose of this chapter is to briefly describe, in chronological fashion, the stages of rehabilitation from referral to discharge of the patient (see Table 5–1).

patient referred

Patients referred for services in the hospital are typically in an acute stage of illness with a recent medical diagnosis or are undergoing diagnostic tests to establish a diagnosis. Exceptions are those with a progressive disorder who only recently have reached the point where communicative skills are significantly affected or patients whose physician works under the premise that speech and language services are in order only when physiological recovery has reached a plateau. The referral information is usually succinct and limited to statements like ". . . 62-year-old female with progressive supranuclear palsy" or ". . . 72-year-old male with aphasia secondary to left cerebrovascular accident." At times the speech/language pathologist may be asked whether referral of a patient is warranted. The procedure should be to review the medical chart, briefly screen the patient, and then to decide, based on this information, whether referral would be beneficial to the patient.

background information

Although some clinicians prefer to see the patient before the chart, the preferable procedure is to first review the medical records. Data contained in the medical record was reviewed in the chapter on evaluation. Included are identifying information; familial, educational, vocational, and medical histories; results of diagnostic procedures; doctor's orders and progress notes; nurses' notes; reports from other rehabilitation services; and discharge summaries from other facilities. Remember that this is a most important data base for establishing a contextual framework for diagnosis and for determining a prognosis. It is worthwhile to record pertinent infor-

TABLE 5-1

Stages of the Rehabilitation Process

A. Referral of patient to speech-language pathologist

B. Collection of contextual background information
   1. Medical chart
      a. Identifying information
      b. Medical, familial, educational, and vocational histories
      c. Results of diagnostic procedures
      d. Doctors' and nurses' notes; progress notes
   2. Discharge summaries from other facilities
   3. Information directly obtained from family and physician

C. Informal assessment
   1. Estimate type and severity of disorder
   2. Identify motor, sensory, and behavioral deficits that affect assessment

D. Evaluation
   1. Standardized tests
   2. Informal measurements

E. Tentative diagnosis and prognosis: Evaluation report

F. Treatment
   1. Provide information and counseling for patient, family, and staff
   2. Decrease environmental demand, increase environmental opportunity, and enhance patient compensatory strategies for communication
   3. Provide direct treatment
      a. Identify patient's abilities and needs
      b. Identify treatment target areas and rationales
      c. Perform task analysis of target areas
      d. Identify patient's behavior within task analysis
      e. Establish performance goals
      f. Determine treatment sequence
      g. Monitor progress

G. Terminate treatment based on evaluation of progress and patient's needs

mation while reviewing the chart since it will be necessary to refer to it when the evaluation report is written. If the patient resides in a nursing home, the information available may be considerably less detailed because patients are frequently admitted directly from their homes without an extensive medical evaluation. In these cases, the attending physician and family should be contacted regarding sources of additional data.

informal assessment

The next step is to informally evaluate the patient. Two specific types of information are sought: (1) an estimate of the type and severity of impairment, and (2) the presence of motor and sensory deficits and emotional problems that may affect formal test performance. The protocol used to assess impairment is brief and tailored to the type of deficit expected from review of the medical records. Generally, the patient is asked to provide a short history of his problem and to provide his name, address, place of employment, hobbies, etc. He also is requested to write identifying information; to name objects in the room, body parts, and articles of clothing; to repeat short sentences; to follow commands; and to read words and sentences. This brief evaluation yields information on orientation, memory, oral expression, auditory comprehension, reading, writing, and speech intelligibility. It can be abbreviated or expanded depending on the patient's deficits. Particular attention also should be paid to compensatory strategies used during the assessment. Does the patient use gestures such as pointing? Does he write answers to questions he cannot produce orally? Does he indicate by gestures (head shaking, hand movements) that he does not understand the question? etc.

Information on sensory and motor impairments is provided in part by the above protocol. For example, does the patient use the nondominant hand to write? Does he gesture with this hand? Does he have difficulty distinguishing visually presented materials? Does he indicate he cannot hear auditorally presented information? Additionally, procedures for assessing visual field deficits, as outlined in the evaluation chapter, are undertaken, if warranted, and if a significant hearing impairment is evident, auditory acuity testing is included in the formal assessment battery to follow. A judgment of emotional status also is made since depression, frustration, anger, etc., may affect test performance.

In summary, four important purposes are served by the informal assessment: (1) estimates of type and severity of communicative impairment aid in test selection, (2) determination of motor and sensory impairment helps predict how tests may need to be adapted for the patient, (3) judgments of emotional stability provide information on whether formal assessment will yield maximal performance, and (4) the establishment of rapport lessens patient anxiety in the formal test situation, particularly if information is provided on the evaluation plan, its purpose, and the approximate time required for its completion.

Assessment of Communicative Skills The informal assessment usually provides sufficient information for selection of appraisal instruments and procedures for formal testing. The results of the tests and other observations are interpreted within the context of the background information to determine a diagnosis. Prognosis is based on the diagnosis and contextual information available. Evaluation and prognosis were discussed in detail earlier. They will not be considered further at this point.

evaluation report

The means by which assessment information is conveyed to the referring source is the evaluation report. Reports of this type, especially in medical settings, are brief. Included in sections are (1) background history which is summarized from medical records and any other sources of information; (2) a statement of clinical observations which describe the patient's alertness, cooperativeness, and apparent motor and sensory deficits; (3) descriptions of the tests administered and results obtained; (4) a tentative diagnosis of the disorder (aphasia, apraxia, dysarthria, confusion) with additional descriptive information, if needed, to convey the full extent of the impairment; and (5) recommendations for treatment, including prognosis for recovery of communicative functioning. The recommendations are prescriptive, indicating the type and frequency of therapy to be provided.

The brevity of the report does not reflect its value in information transmission. Although some patients may receive all rehabilitation from diagnosis to treatment termination within a single hospital (e.g., Veterans Administration), more commonly they will be transferred one or more times. For example, Gibson (1974) found that of 383 cases of stroke admitted to hospitals in Monroe County, New York, 35 percent were discharged home, 28 were discharged to other institutions, and 37 percent died. Facilities to which patients were transferred included 15 different nursing homes, 5 church homes for the aged, 2 hospital extended-care facilities, a county chronic disease hospital, a Veterans Administration hospital, and several other rehabilitation facilities. It would also be anticipated that some of the patients discharged to nursing and rehabilitation facilities would ultimately be discharged home, and some patients discharged home would eventually be admitted to nursing facilities or return to the hospital. It is, therefore, important that the evaluation reports and treatment records provide a succinct description of the initial problems, the treatment applied, the effects of therapy, and status at discharge.

In addition to initial evaluation reports, patient contact, interim, and final case reports contain assessment information. Patient contact records can take more than one form. They may be a simple descriptive note recorded in the progress notes or be more structured. Many facilities now use Problem-Oriented Medical Records (POMR) which include SOAP categories. SOAP stands for Subjective, Objective, Assessment and Plans (Bouchard and Shane, 1977). In terms of POMR contact records, subjective information would involve description of the patient's cooperativeness, attitude, complaints, and so on, observed during the treatment session. Objective information includes a statement of performance on the tasks administered. The assessment section reports progress in objective terms, and the plans section is a description of the next planned activities in the treatment of the patient.

Background information, goals of treatment, procedures applied, progress to date, and a plan for additional therapy is included in an interim report. These reports are typically reserved for patients undergoing long-term treatment and who are being evaluated at extended intervals by the entire rehabilitation team. Final reports include the same sections, but a discharge plan is substituted for the section dealing with additional proposed treatment. The final report, then, is a summary of all activities carried out with the patient from initial referral to termination of treatment at that facility. It contains information from the initial evaluation, therapy contact reports, and interim reports and is forwarded when information regarding the patient is requested.

treatment

Regardless of the type of neurogenic communication disorder, the speech-language pathologist performs three functions: provides information and emotional support, reduces environmental demands and increases environmental opportunity for communication, and directs treatment towards specific disordered communicative processes. The first two functions will be considered together since they heavily overlap and will be preceded by a discussion of the psychoemotional problems of the neurogenic patient and his family.

Counseling and the Communication Process An increasing body of research suggests that the adjustment of the patient and family to brain damage has an important impact on expected recovery. The adjustments are not simply to the communicative disorder, but to long-term changes in the social, financial, and emotional structure of the family. Perhaps the most comprehensive description of psychological reactions of aphasic patients is provided by Eisenson (1973). He emphasized the role of premorbid personality in determining the patient's individual reactions to aphasia. However he noted that aphasics, as a group, tend to experience similar emotional reactions—"fear, loneliness, lowered self-esteem and defensive concern for the thoughts of others" (p. 89). The reactions to a life-changing situation, such as serious illness or injury or imminent death, are so universal that a four-part pattern has been posited as the "... behavioral expression of an ongoing process of cognitive and emotional incorporation of trauma leading to readjustment" (Falek and Britton, 1974, p. 5). The pattern described consists of (1) shock and denial, (2) anxiety, (3) anger and/or guilt, and (4) depression. Denial is a refusal, at least for a brief period, to accept the situation as it is and is followed by anxiety as the patient attempts to deal intellectually with the problem. Anger and/or guilt arise from the patient's failure and frustration and leads to depression when frustration becomes habituated. The depression is characterized by a feeling that there is a lack of meaning and a sense of isolation. Depression is a common theme in aphasic patients' accounts of their stroke and recovery (e.g., Ritchie, 1961). It will be expected that this pattern of reactions will be repeated a number of times by the patient, hopefully with decreasing intensity, and will ultimately lead to an adjustment to residual deficits.

The need to deal effectively with predictable emotional reactions is paramount to the rehabilitation effort. There is little reason to believe that a patient who has not come to recognize the residuals of brain damage will be sufficiently motivated to participate actively in the long-term effort. Hyman (1969), for example, investigated the effects of stroke patients' attitudes toward illness and premorbid life situations on motivation and functional improvement in rehabilitation. Physical therapists rated motivation and nurses, occupational therapists, and physical therapists rated functional improvement. Hyman noted, among other findings, that the stigma of stroke and the feelings of social isolation and dependency adversely affected motivation and functional improvement.

The family also undergoes emotional changes. Turnblom and Myers (1952) observed that:

> . . . the family faces problems of equal concern [to those of the patient]. A former healthy and independent member, possibly the breadwinner, suddenly becomes highly dependent. Feelings of pity and hostility, shame and guilt may all develop, depending on the emotional maturity of the individuals. These feelings easily become intensified by the added financial burden, uncertainty as to the length and type of treatment, ignorance of limitations, precautions and prognosis, and by indecisiveness over the individual's own role. These emotional disturbances in the family will quickly be reflected in the patient's outlook and motivation. (p. 393)

Biorn-Hansen (1957) noted that one of the most frequent family problems was a change in the role of the patient, including a shift in responsibilities and an altered relationship with the spouse and children. The spouse may assume responsibilities that he or she is hesitant to give up as the patient improves; unsatisfactory sexual relations may arise from impotency and rejection; the patient may become overprotected or rejected, feel incapable of satisfactorily participating in parenting, and become increasingly dependent in the presence of the long-term illness. Similarly Malone (1969), in 25 interviews, identified problems expressed by the families of aphasic patients. These included (1) role changes, (2) irritability, (3) guilt feelings, (4) altered social life, (5) financial problems, (6) job neglect, (7) health problems, (8) oversolicitousness or rejection of the patient, and (9) changes in parenting. What might be concluded is that both the family and patient must be beneficiaries of counseling directed toward the communicative impairment and the psychosocial and emotional responses to the illness. Since rehabilitation personnel are involved in this process, they too must be provided with information regarding the communicative impairment and its impact on the family and patient.

Counseling the Patient A frequent assumption is that the neurogenic patient is fully aware of his predicament. Unfortunately, the information is typically provided at a time when he is least able to understand, remember, or ask questions. It is a reasonable belief that the speech-language pathologist, through testing and observation, is well qualified to provide information and counseling. Following evaluation, the patient should be informed of the nature of the illness, the sensory, motor, behavioral, and communicative consequences of the neurogenic lesion, and the proposed rehabilitation plan. He also should be advised that the clinician is aware of the emotional reactions (anxiety, fear, frustration, depression) the patient may feel in response to the illness, that they are not unexpected, and that the staff will be available to discuss these reactions when he feels the need to consider them. Discussion should not be forced unless it becomes patently clear that the patient's continued avoidance of dealing with these emotional reactions has a significant adverse effect on rehabilitation. One caution is that information directly related to the medical diagnosis, the medical treatment of the disorder, and premorbid psychiatric conditions should clearly be referred to the patient's physician and that questions related to vocational potential and financial difficulties should be referred to other professionals more directly concerned with these matters.

Counseling the Family   Much of the information provided to the family relates directly to the communicative disorder. The type and severity of communicative impairment, the neurological basis for the disorder, the prognosis for significant return of speech and language functioning, and the goals and procedures of treatment (if warranted) are topics to be discussed during the course of rehabilitation.

There is some reason to believe that the spouse's estimate of residual communicative ability may be different from that of the clinician's. Helmick, Watamori, and Palmer (1976) found a significant negative correlation between spouses' ratings of communicative ability on a modified form of the Functional Communication Profile and Porch Index of Communicative Ability scores, whereas a highly significant positive correlation was noted for clinician ratings and the Porch scores. Helmick et al. concluded that spouses had a significant tendency to judge the aphasic's communication as less impaired compared to judgments by a speech-language pathologist. However Holland (1977) argued that aphasia tests, such as the PICA, are perhaps better measures of language than of communication and that the patient's communication observed in the clinical setting may not be a valid indication of his or her abilities in the context of more typical speaking situations. In counseling, it is best to convey to the family member that the patient's communicative effectiveness will be at least partially context-dependent.

The clinician also provides information on how communication can most effectively be carried out with the patient. Written information may aid this process. Communication suggestions for the aphasic patient are provided in Table 5–2. They should be altered or expanded to meet the patient's situation and disorder. Their similarity to the characteristics of the stimuli used in treatment is not happenstance.

TABLE 5-2

How to Talk Effectively to Adult Aphasic Patients

1. Speak slowly.
2. Allow the patient ample time to respond.
3. Use short simple sentences.
4. Remember that the patient may have a short attention span.
5. In most cases use high frequency words familiar to the patient.
6. Provide situational cues so that the patient is able to anticipate the nature of the conversation.
7. Speak in a manner consistent with conventional syntactic and semantic rules.
8. Do not speak loudly to the patient.
9. Do not correct the patient unless he or she desires to be corrected and allow the patient to speak for him/herself unless he or she requests aid.
10. Ask questions which have yes or no answers.
11. Do not require that the patient communicate with large groups of people or in noisy surroundings.
12. Be aware that the patient may perform better on some tasks when they are presented in isolation rather than in series with other tasks.
13. Use meaningful gestures and facial expressions liberally.
14. Repeat or rephrase a stimulus when a patient does not understand it after the first presentation.
15. Speak appropriately to aphasic patients with hearing losses. In other words, articulate carefully, don't shout, use gestures, get the patient's attention before speaking, and face him or her while speaking.
16. Convey a calm, reassuring, and encouraging attitude to the patient.
17. Do not speak to the patient as if he or she were a child.

Adapted from Flowers, C. How to talk effectively to adult aphasic patients. *J. Minn. Speech Hearing Association*, 1973, *12*, 26–30. Reprinted by permission.

Information about the patient's and family's responses to the disorder should be conveyed in an atmosphere conducive to an open expression of concerns. It is wise, in most cases, for the family to be counseled without the patient present. However there are situations where the clinician may judge a joint meeting to be most beneficial.

If operative in the clinical setting, patient-family interactive groups are excellent for establishing stable lines of communication with rehabilitation personnel for the purpose of dealing with the emotional responses to the patient's illness. These groups have included patients (e.g., Blackman and Tureen, 1948), family members (e.g., Turnblom and Myers, 1952), and patients and families (Redinger, Forster, Dolphin, Godduhn, and Weisinger, 1971); have generally been directed through a joint effort of speech-language pathologist, psychologist, or psychiatrist; and have been reported to be successful at dealing with psychosocial and emotional aspects of rehabilitation.

Also of value for continuing support for patients are stroke clubs. According to the National Easter Seal Society (1972), the purposes of a stroke club are (1) to unite stroke victims for the purpose of aiding each other, (2) to instruct stroke victims and their families regarding the nature of strokes and the means for overcoming handicaps generated by them, and (3) to give hope to new stroke patients and to encourage them to improve themselves" (p. 1). Suggestions for organizing a club are provided by the American

Heart Association (1974). Perhaps the major distinction between clubs and aphasia groups is that in clubs the patients supervise and organize the activities. Clubs have proven of significant value in providing information, recreation, and socialization and in maintaining continuing contact with rehabilitation personnel following termination of treatment.

The success of counseling is dependent on patient and family acceptance of the clinicians's judgment and the information provided. Two examples may help to clarify this point. An electrical engineer suffered an occlusion of the left middle cerebral artery and was left severely aphasic and hemiplegic. During the six-month course of treatment, the hemiplegia improved to the point where he could care for himself independently, but his communication skills were very limited. The patient was depressed and suicidal. The neurologist referred him to another speech-language pathology center for reevaluation. Testing confirmed a severe aphasia. Discussion with the patient's wife revealed that his depression could be attributed to his belief that the aphasia would resolve through continued work on reading and writing exercises provided at his discharge from the rehabilitation program and that he would be able to return to his previous employment. The patient and spouse were counseled, individually and then together, that only limited improvement in communication skills with or without treatment could be expected and that a return to a comparable premorbid employment was not possible. The patient appeared relieved since he felt that the failure of the aphasia to resolve was because he did not work hard or long enough on the materials provided and that this in turn required his wife to seek employment outside the home. Referral to a vocational rehabilitation counselor resulted in employment with the same company, albeit in a markedly reduced capacity. At last report the patient and his wife had made an excellent adjustment to the residual effects of the illness.

A young logger was involved in a car-truck accident which left him with bilateral traumatic brain damage. His motor and language skills recovered, but he remained confused with significantly impaired judgment. The discharge plan recommended placement in a nearby neuropsychiatric hospital. The patient's wife was informed of the reasons for this decision. However she was convinced from limited visits with the patient that his problems would be minimized in a familiar home environment. Two weeks later she returned and requested neuropsychiatric placement. Upon return home the patient had on several occasions taken the car without his wife's knowledge, driven to nearby cities, and become lost. She only learned of his whereabouts when someone came to his aid and informed her of his location. The patient also became confused regarding the location of the bathroom and toileted wherever it was convenient and did not always recognize his children. The highly structured environment of the neuropsychiatric hospital where he was admitted allowed the patient to operate with relatively little difficulty, and he was close enough for the family to visit.

Providing Information to Rehabilitation Staff Information is provided to the staff in several ways. First, the evaluation report communicates the characteristics of the patient's speech and language disorder to the physician, nurses, and other rehabilitative staff. It should be supplemented, if at all possible, by direct discussion of the patient in the context of a rehabilitation team meeting or on an individual basis. Two excellent means of providing communication suggestions to primary caregivers (nurses, nurses' aids, orderlies), and visitors to the patient are to type them on 4 X 6 cards and to post them at the patient's bedside and in the nursing file. The nursing file includes the tasks to be performed for each patient during each nursing shift and is reviewed at each shift change. Visitors usually make every effort to follow the suggestions posted which facilitates the types of long-standing personal interactions so needed by the patient during the early stages of recovery or at the point in a progressive degenerative disease when the patient feels the greatest need to communicate. It is worth repeating that the role of the speech-language pathologist as an information source begins at referral and continues until rehabilitation has been completed or the patient is discharged.

fostering communicative interaction

The information source function of the clinician overlaps with the task of reducing the communicative demands on the patient. For example, informing the staff that the patient understands short questions if repeated and presented slowly and that the patient reliably responds "yes" and "no" with head gestures allows him or her to choose meals, to decide on the activity to participate in during a recreational period, and to indicate the need for toileting. The environment should be structured so that the most immediate needs of the patient are at hand and do not need to be requested. Glasses, hearing aid, dentures, walker, water, paper and pencil, bathrobe, tobacco products, radio, and other frequently used items should be available at bedside. If there is a question whether the patient can obtain a needed item due to neuromuscular impairment, trial runs on obtaining objects are carried out. A fixed schedule is important. If the patient is aware of when specific tasks, such as toileting and feeding, will be performed, he or she does not need to request them.

Coupled to information transmission and reducing communicative demands is the enhancement of compensatory strategies used by the patient to convey information. The repertoire of residual skills should be examined. If single-word communication supplemented by gestures is efficient for the patient, then this should be the initial system used. Alternate modes are particularly important at this point in rehabilitation. If verbal communication is not possible, then writing or communication boards are the most logical choices as alternative modes. Any and all combinations of verbal, written, gestural, and gesture-assisted communication should be considered.

The point to be made is that the information provided to the family and rehabilitation staff maximize communicative access to the patient. Capitalizing on compensatory strategies supplemented by other modes provides the patient with access to his or her communicative environment.

The difficulties inherent in this generation of two-way communication varies with the neurogenic condition. For the severely dysarthric or apractic patient with reasonably intact auditory comprehension, an expressive strategy needs to be developed, but this is relatively easy compared to devising systems for the patient with severe comprehension and expression problems. In some cases, such as advanced dementia, the patient may be unable to utilize any communicative system and is relegated to the lowest level of nursing care—anticipation of all care needs.

The use of strategies to allow access to and from the patient does not guarantee that communicative interaction will take place. There must be a fostering of environmental opportunity for the patient to use residual skills in meaningful situations. Opportunities do not necessarily have to be manufactured since the hospital routine includes interaction with staff and family members who, if adequately informed of the patient's communicative limitations, will actively engage the patient in conversation. It is helpful, however, to interview the patient and family to identify activities that can be built into the patient's schedule and that involve speaking partners who value the patient's participation. For example, regular visits by volunteers who have similar interests can be arranged, coworkers can be invited to see the patient, and hospital recreational activities can be scheduled. If a recreational therapist is employed in the facility, referral to this resource is in order.

therapy for specific disorders

The third in the triad of functions performed by the clinician is therapy directed toward improving specific speech and language disorders. The philosophy espoused here is that direct treatment is an eclectic attempt to improve upon the communication system established early in the post-onset period in the case of acute brain damage, or to develop and maintain maximal performance in light of residual abilities in progressive disorders. In other words, the clinician attempts to establish, to improve the efficiency, and/or to maintain the integrity of the patient's communicative abilities.

Whether direct therapy is undertaken is determined by the prognosis. Prognostic indicators aid in determining *what* services will be provided, not *if* they will be provided. Information giving and fostering communicative interaction are clinical services available to the patient regardless of prognosis. It is best to be conservative when making decisions about direct therapy. If the prognosis is guarded, a trial period of therapy should be implemented.

Even for this limited effort, however, performance goals should be set, and if not met, therapy should be terminated.

Direct therapy includes a definable series of tasks. The tasks are completed regardless of the diagnosis.

Identify Patient's Abilities and Needs Results of the assessment battery are reexamined to identify reading, writing, auditory comprehension, speech, mathematics, "functional" communication, etc. levels of functioning as the first step. This data should already be available from the evaluation but now is used to aid in therapy planning rather than in determining a diagnosis. At the same time, the patient's communication needs and whatever strategies are used to meet these needs are identified and recorded. One useful tool to accomplish this purpose is to maintain a log of communication engaged in and problems encountered (Figure 5–1). The log can be completed by a family member, the clinician, or the patient, if he is able. As a minimum requirement, the log must contain a *representative sampling* from a number of situations since communication needs and success are influenced by context. For example, a patient will experience considerably more success at explaining a calculation error in the checkbook to a sympathetic family member than to a bank teller. For the patient with a minimal impairment, the log may include only situations where difficulty is experienced. The log should be supplemented by interviewing the patient, family members, coworkers, hospital staff, etc. as to what communication needs the patient must meet in the hospital, home, work, and other environments. As a result of reexamining evaluation data and determining communication needs, an estimate of how closely residual skills fulfill needs can be made to serve as a departure point for identifying target areas for direct therapy.

Identify Treatment Target Areas and Rationales What communication needs will be addressed in direct therapy is a joint decision of patient and clinician and will vary as a function of diagnosis and personal circumstances. For the severely apractic patient in a nursing home, the primary need may be a gestural communication system; for the mildly aphasic patient returning to employment in a store, it may be improving calculation skills; for the patient with a progressive neurological disorder and dysarthria, it may be improved speech intelligibility. There are typically more needs than can be treated at one time. Therefore, priorities must logically be established. There must also be a clear definition of rationales for the targeted treatment areas clearly understood and agreed upon by the patient.

Perform Task Analysis of Target Areas A task analysis is a determination of what skills are required for the performance of a specific activity. For example, in constructing a shopping list within a defined budget, tasks

LOG OF COMMUNICATIVE ACTIVITY DURING DAILY EVENTS

PATIENT R.C.   CLINIC NUMBER 80-0847   DIAGNOSIS Aphasia

DATE 8/18/80   INFORMANT Wife

ROUTINE: MEALTIMES, TELEPHONING, SHOPPING, DISCIPLINING CHILDREN, CHECKBOOK, ETC.

NON-ROUTINE: DINING OUT, DOCTOR'S OFFICE, WEEKEND EVENTS, EMERGENCY SITUATIONS

TIME	ACTIVITY	PATIENT COMMUNICATION (INCLUDING MODALITIES USED)	WITH WHOM	PROBLEMS (DESCRIBE)
8:00	Breakfast	Asks children what they want prepared for breakfast. Uses gestures and verbal expression.	Children- Mark and Cindy	Has difficulty understanding children's response. Must be repeated several times.
8:30	Telephone	Wife calls to tell patient time of his doctor's appointment.	Wife	Message must be repeated. Patient writes time on memo pad.
9:00	Visit by exterminator.	Patient tells exterminator that roaches have been seen in kitchen. Gestures to places they have been seen. Writes check to pay for services.	Exterminator	Patient has difficulty writing name of company. Signs check and fills out monetary amount without company name.
10:00	Hospital Volunteer	Talks with patient regarding recreation activities. Uses gestures and verbal expression.	Patient	Has difficulty understanding patient's questions regarding times that bingo will be played. Patient upset by inability to communicate information.
2:00	Disciplining children	Tells children (using gestures) to be quiet so that he can sleep.	Children	Children continue to talk loudly. Patient not able to enforce sufficient quiet to sleep. Goes to his room.
3:00	Telephone	Solicitor calls to investigate patient's interest in re-roofing home.	Salesman	Patient hangs up without responding.
5:00	Supper	Reads recipe to prepare meal.	—	Patient has difficulty following steps of the recipe.
6:00	Reads paper.	—	—	Specific information from stories cannot be recalled.

FIGURE 5-1 Log of Communicative Activity During Daily Events

would include identifying and writing the list of needed items, recording and adding up the cost of each item, and comparing the total to the budget limitation. Similar analyses are required for each communication need targeted for direct treatment.

Identify Patient's Behavior within the Task Analysis The next step is to determine the patient's behavior within the task analysis. That is, how well can the patient perform the tasks encompassed within a communicative activity. For example, if the activity is telephoning, can the patient find names and numbers in the directory, dial seven digit numbers, ask for information to obtain names and numbers not in the directory, and so forth. Additional evaluation beyond the assessment battery results may be needed since the primary purpose of the evaluation was to identify the type and severity of the disorder and not the performance of the patient on all possible communication tasks.

Generate Treatment Goals Goals are established based upon the patient's expected performance. Initial and interim goals should be structured to accomplish long-term objectives. If Amer-Ind were used with a severely apractic patient, for example, initial goals might include recognition, execution, and retrieval of a preset number of signs, interim goals, the use of these gestures in a controlled context, and long term goals, the use of the code in spontaneous conversation at a level approximating propositional speech. Goals are set for specific time periods that vary as a function of setting and funding source. Medicare requires recertification at 30 day periods; many university facilities set goals for a semester or quarter. Goals should generally be considered tentative until progress can be monitored and the patient's performance more accurately gauged for given time spans.

Determine Treatment Sequence A large number of materials are available for constructing treatment sequences for aphasic (Keith, 1971, 1977; Longerich, 1965; Stryker, 1975; Taylor and Marks, 1959; Traendly, 1977) and apractic (Hill, 1978; Rosenbek, 1978) patients. Patients with dysarthria may require mechanical or surgical intervention (e.g., Arnold, 1962; Gonzalez and Aronson, 1970; Johns and Salyer, 1978) to develop structural-functional substitutes for immobilized musculature at laryngeal or velopharyngeal valves before treatment sequences utilizing physiological-instrumental (e.g., Netsell and Cleeland, 1973; Netsell and Daniel, 1979) and behavioral (Darley, et al., 1975; Rosenbek and LaPointe, 1978) therapy are employed.

This is the point in direct therapy where many of the treatment methods discussed in Chapter Four are relevant. As part of this task, cues, prompts, and stimulus attributes are explored to identify which, if used individually or in combination, maximize performance. Base-10 forms are particularly helpful for this purpose. After informal conversation with the patient during which the most influential variables are isolated, series of ten items can be presented over as many as ten trials to determine percentile performance as a function of the variable combinations. Brookshire (1978) recommended that correct responses at the beginning of a treatment activity should be between 60 and 80 percent and that the difficulty of the task should be increased when correct responses exceed 90 percent. Both "correct" performance and task difficulty are at least partially definitional. If dichotomous scoring is used, percentages are based on the total number of correct responses out of a group of specified items. If PICA scoring is used, success is defined qualitatively. Difficulty is defined by increasing the complexity of the task or by reducing the cues and prompts used to aid performance. This step then consists of constructing a sequence of materials to address particular communication needs and then pretesting the levels of the sequence to determine the point at which performance is partially but not completely successful where therapy begins.

Monitoring Progress As part of the process of determining and implementing a therapy sequence, records of performance over repeated sessions are maintained to monitor progress. Several tasks should be included in each session and feedback provided as a contingency of successful or unsuccessful performance and as objective evidence of progress toward stated and agreed upon goals. Since therapy is usually limited to several hours per week, a home program of activities needs to be structured that is similar to the tasks employed in therapy. These can be evaluated and considered in determinations of progress. Whether progress is sufficient to merit continued therapy is relative and judgmental. No absolute rules can be offered since small gains may be adequate reason for continued treatment of a severely involved patient but not a mildly impaired patient.

treatment termination

Completion of rehabilitation and termination of the program should come as no surprise to the patient. Information provided at the outset prepares him or her for the program that subsequently transpires. Throughout the treatment period, feedback in the form of a graphic display of progress and appropriate comments regarding the significance of the improvement is usually adequate to the task of informing him or her of when termination is appropriate. There appears to be agreement (Warren, 1976) that, as part of the termination decision, the patient should be counseled that treatment will soon end and that it should be viewed as a positive event since rehabilitation has been completed. It should be noted, however, that termination may be beyond the control of the patient and clinician due to the unaffordable costs of services or the distance from the rehabilitation site.

The rehabilitation process has a number of overlapping and identifiable steps. Upon referral, review of patient medical records and informal assessment identify the skills to be evaluated and the sensory, motor, and behavioral deficits that affect appraisal. Test instruments are chosen to determine the type and severity of the communication deficits, and a diagnosis is established by placing formal evaluation test results into the context of background information. By reviewing relevant data available from test results and medical records, a decision on prognosis and treatment program is made. The diagnosis, prognosis, treatment plan, and means by which communication with the patient is maximized are transmitted to the patient, family, and rehabilitation personnel. An ongoing dialogue with the patient and family is initiated to help them in dealing with emotional responses to the disorders produced by the nervous system impairment. Direct therapy, if warranted, addresses specific deficits and is geared toward establishing and improving upon a functional communication system or developing skills that will aid the patient in maintaining speech and language abilities when faced with a progressive degenerative neurogenic disease. Termination of treatment is based on knowledge of progress toward reasonable and agreed-upon goals and the prognosis for recovery. During the course of the rehabilitation effort, diagnosis, prognosis, treatment plan, and counseling concerns are reevaluated and altered as new information becomes available and new problems are identified.

○ CONCLUSIONS

It is difficult to summarize the many topics addressed in this text—perhaps none is necessary. An effort has been made to provide basic information on neurogenic communication disorders, the tasks to be performed in their rehabilitation, and the instruments and procedures available for this purpose. Several points have been stressed. First, rehabilitation must be predicated on data-based research findings that provide the rationale for the treatment applied and for the hypotheses generated. Second, neurogenic communication disorders are sufficiently unique and the clinician-patient interaction sufficiently complex to preclude generating a prescriptive treatment paradigm for the next patient who crosses the clinic's threshhold. Each patient and his or her problems must be considered individually. Finally, the rehabilitation process involves more than the patient and clinician. The family is affected significantly by the patient's problems, and brain damage produces multiple disorders that require the expertise of other rehabilitation personnel. All must be actively involved during the course of rehabilitation.

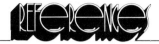

Ajuriaguerra, J. de, and Tissot, R. Some aspects of language in various forms of senile dementia (comparisons with language in childhood). In E. Lenneberg and E. Lenneberg (Eds.), *Foundations of language development* (Vol. 1). New York: Academic Press, 1975.

Albert, M., Sparks, R., and Helm, N. Melodic intonation therapy for aphasia. *Arch. Neurol.*, 1973, 29, 130–131.

Alpers, B., & Mancall, E. *Essentials of the neurological examination.* Philadelphia: F. A. Davis, 1971.

American Heart Association. *A guideline for American Heart Association stroke clubs.* Austin: American Heart Association Texas Affiliate, 1974.

Anderson, T. P., Bourestom, N., and Greenberg, F. *Rehabilitation predictors in completed stroke: Final report.* Minneapolis: American Rehabilitation Foundation, 1970.

Appel, F., and Appel, E. Intracranial variation in the weight of the human brain. *Human Biol.*, 1942, *14*, 48–68. (a)

Appel, F., and Appel, E., Intracranial variation in the weight of the human brain. *Human Biol.*, 1942, *14*, 235–250. (b)

Arenberg, D. Cognition and aging: Verbal learning, memory and problem solving. In C. Eisdorfer & M. Lawton (Eds.), *The psychology of adult development and aging.* Washington, D.C.: American Psychological Association, 1973.

Arnold, G. Vocal rehabilitation of paralytic dysphonia: IX. Technique of intracordal injection. *Arch. Otolaryng.*, 1962, *76*, 358–368.

Baker, N., and Holland, A. Aphasic comprehension of related statements. In A. Holland, *Psycholinguistic and behavioral variables underlying recovery from aphasia.* Washington, D.C.: Social and Rehabilitation Service, Department of Health, Education, and Welfare, 1971.

Baptista, A. G. Aspects of cerebral circulation. In H. E. Himwich (Ed.), *Brain metabolism and cerebral disorders.* New York: Spectrum Publications, 1976.

Barker, M., and Lawson, J. Nominal aphasia in dementia. *Brit. J. Psychiat.*, 1968, *114*, 1351–1356.

Barrett, J. *Gerontological pathology.* Springfield, Ill.: Chas. C Thomas, 1972.

Barton, M., Maruszewski, M., and Urrea, D. Variation of stimulus context and its effect on word-finding ability in aphasics. *Cortex,* 1969, *5*, 351–365.

Basso, A., Capitani, E., and Vignolo, L. Influence of rehabilitation on language skills in aphasic patients: A controlled study. *Arch. Neurol.*, 1979, *36*, 190–196.

Bay, E. The classification of disorders of speech. *Cortex,* 1967, *3*, 26–31.

Bell, K., and Goepfert, H. Rehabilitation of head and neck cancer patients to deglutinate. *Tejas,* 1977, *2*, 3–5.

Benton, A. *Benton revised visual retention test.* New York: Psychological Corporation, 1974.

Benton, A. Problems of test construction in the field of aphasia. *Cortex,* 1967, *3,* 32–58.

Berlin, C. On melodic intonation therapy for aphasia by R. W. Sparks & A. L. Holland. *J. Speech Hearing Dis.,* 1976, *41,* 298–300.

Berman, M., and Peele, L. Self-generated cues: A method of aiding aphasic and apractic patients. *J. Speech Hearing Dis.,* 1967, *32,* 372–376.

Berry, R. Pathology of dementia. In J. G. Howells (Ed.), *Modern perspectives in the psychiatry of old age.* New York: Brunner/Mazel, 1975.

Berry, W., Darley, F., Aronson, A., and Goldstein, N. Dysarthria in Wilson's disease. *J. Speech Hearing Res.,* 1974, *17,* 169–183.

Beyn, E., and Shokhor-Trotskaya, M. The preventive method of speech rehabilitation. *Cortex,* 1966, *2,* 96–108.

Biorn-Hansen, V., Social and emotional aspects of aphasia. *J. Speech Hearing Dis.,* 1957, *22,* 53–59.

Blackman, N., and Tureen, L. Aphasia—A psychosomatic approach in rehabilitation. *Tran. Amer. Neurol. Assoc.,* 1948, *73,* 193–196.

Bloom, W., and Fawcett, D. *A textbook of histology* (10th ed.). Philadelphia: Saunders, 1975.

Blumstein, S. *A phonological investigation of aphasic speech.* The Hague: Mouton, 1973.

Bogen, J., and Bogen, G. Wernicke's region—Where is it? *Ann. NY Acad. Med.,* 1977, *280,* 834–843.

Boller, F., and Vignolo, L. Latent sensory aphasia in hemisphere damaged patients: An experimental study with the token test. *Brain,* 1966, *89,* 815–830.

Bollinger, R., and Stout, C. Response contingent small step treatment: Performance-based communication intervention. *J. Speech Hearing Dis.,* 1976, *41,* 40–51.

Bondareff, W. Morphology of the aging nervous system. In J. E. Birren (Ed.), *Handbook of aging and the individual: Psychological and biological aspects.* Chicago: University of Chicago Press, 1959.

Borkowski, J., Benton, A., and Spreen, O. Word fluency and brain damage. *Neuropsychologia,* 1967, *5,* 135–140.

Botwinick, J. *Cognitive processes in maturity and old age.* New York: Springer, 1967.

Botwinick, J. Geropsychology. *Annual Rev. Psych.,* 1970, *21,* 239–272.

Bouchard, M., and Shane, H. Use of the problem-oriented medical record in the speech and hearing profession. *ASHA,* 1977, *19,* 829–833.

Brain, R. Henry Head: The man and his ideas. *Brain,* 1961, *84,* 561–566.

Brody, H. Organization of the cerebral cortex. III. A study of aging in human cerebral cortex. *J. Comp. Neurol.* 1955, *102,* 511–556.

Brody, H. Structural changes in the aging nervous system. *Inter. Topics Geront.,* 1970, *7,* 9–21.

Brody, H., and Vyayashankar, N. Anatomical changes in the nervous system. In C. Finch & L. Hayflick (Eds.), *The handbook of the biology of aging.* New York: Van Nostrand Reinhold, 1977.

Brookshire, R. Speech pathology and the experimental analysis of behavior. *J. Speech Hearing Dis.*, 1967, *32*, 215–227.

Brookshire, R. Effects of delay of reinforcement on probability learning by aphasic subjects. *J. Speech Hearing Res.*, 1971, *14*, 92–105.(a)

Brookshire, R. Effects of trial time and inter-trial interval on naming by aphasic subjects. *J. Commun. Dis.*, 1971, 289–301. (b)

Brookshire, R. Effects of task difficulty on the naming performance of aphasic subjects. *J. Speech Hearing Res.*, 1972, *15*, 551–558.

Brookshire, R. *An introduction to aphasia* (2nd ed.). Minneapolis: BRK Publishers, 1978.

Brown, J. Some clinical aspects of aphasia. *Ann. Otol., Rhinol, Laryng.*, 1960, *69*, 1214–1222.

Butfield, E., and Zangwill, O. Re-education in aphasia: A review of 70 cases. *J. Neurol., Neurosurg., Psychiat.*, 1946, *9*, 75–79.

Butters, N., Rosen, J., and Stein, D. Recovery of behavioral functions after sequential ablation of the frontal lobes of monkeys. In D. Stein, J. Rosen, & N. Butters (Eds.), *Plasticity and recovery of function in the central nervous system.* New York: Academic Press, 1974.

Caramazza, A., & Zurif, E. *Language acquisition and language breakdown: Parallels and divergences.* Baltimore, Md.: Johns Hopkins University Press, 1978.

Carson, D., Carson, F., and Tikofsky, R. On learning characteristics of the adult aphasic. *Cortex*, 1968, *4*, 92–112.

Chafetz, M., Bernstein, N., Sharpe, W., & Schwab, R. Short-term group therapy of patients with Parkinson's disease. *New Engl. J. Med.*, 1955, *253*, 961–964.

Chapey, R. Assessment of language disorders. In R. Chapey (Ed.), *Language intervention strategies in adult aphasia.* Baltimore, Md.: Williams and Wilkins 1981.

Chapey, R. The relationship between divergent and convergent semantic behavior in aphasia. *Arch. Phys. Med. Rehab.*, 1977, *58*, 357–362.

Chapey, R. Divergent semantic intervention. In R. Chapey (Ed.), *Language intervention strategies in adult aphasia.* Baltimore, Md.: Williams & Wilkins, 1981.

Chen, L., "Talking hands" for aphasic stroke patients. *Geriatrics*, 1968, *34*, 145–148.

Chen, L. Manual communication by combined alphabet and gestures. *Arch. Phys. Med. Rehab.*, 1971, *52*, 381–384.

Chusid, J. *Correlative neuroanatomy and functional neurology* (14th ed.). Los Altos, Calif.: Lange Medical Publications, 1970.

Cochran, M. *Conversational prompting.* Veterans Administration Workshop, Temple, Texas, 1980.

Collins, M. The minor hemisphere: Round table discussion. In R. Brookshire (Ed.), *Clinical aphasiology conference proceedings 1976.* Minneapolis: BRK Publishers, 1976.

Corlew, M., and Nation, J. Characteristics of visual stimuli and naming performance in aphasic adults. *Cortex*, 1975, *11*, 186–191.

Costello, J. Programmed instruction. *J. Speech Hearing Dis.*, 1977, *42*, 3–28.

Craik, F. Age differences in human memory. In J. Birren and K. Schaie (Eds.), *Handbook of the psychology of aging.* New York: Van Nostrand Reinhold, 1977.

Culton, G. Spontaneous recovery from aphasia. *J. Speech Hearing Res.*, 1969, *12*, 825–832.

Culton, G. Reaction to age as a factor in chronic aphasia in stroke patients. *J. Speech Hearing Dis.*, 1971, *36*, 563–564.

Cummings, J., Benson, D., Walsh, M., and Levine, H. Left-to-right transfer of language dominance: A case study. *Neurology*, 1979, *29*, 1547–1550.

Czvik, P. The application of an auditory approach using non-variable materials in the treatment of aphasia: Two case studies. In R. Brookshire (Ed.), *Clinical aphasiology conference proceedings 1976.* Minneapolis: BRK Publishers, 1976.

Darley, F. *Diagnosis and appraisal of communication disorders.* Englewood Cliffs, N.J.: Prentice-Hall, 1964.

Darley, F. The efficacy of language rehabilitation in aphasia. *J. Speech Hearing Dis.*, 1972, *37*, 3–21.

Darley, F. Treatment of acquired aphasia. In W. Friedlander (Ed.), *Advances in neurology*, (Vol. 7). New York: Raven Press, 1975.

Darley, F. Maximizing input to the aphasic patient: A review of research. In R. Brookshire (Ed.), *Clinical aphasiology conference proceedings 1976.* Minneapolis: BRK Publishers, 1976.

Darley, F. (Ed.). *Evaluation of appraisal techniques in speech and language pathology.* Reading, Mass.: Addison-Wesley, 1979.

Darley, F., Aronson, A., and Brown, J. Clusters of deviant speech dimensions in the dysarthrias. *J. Speech Hearing Res.*, 1969, *12*, 462–496. (a)

Darley, F., Aronson, A., and Brown, J. Differential diagnostic patterns of dysarthria. *J. Speech Hearing Res.*, 1969, *12*, 246–269. (b)

Darley, F., Aronson, A., and Brown, J. *Motor speech disorders.* Philadelphia: Saunders, 1975.

Darley, F., Brown, J., and Goldstein, N. Dysarthria in multiple sclerosis. *J. Speech Hearing Res.*, 1972, *15*, 229–245.

Darley, F., and Spriestersbach, D. *Diagnostic methods in speech pathology* (2nd ed.). New York: Harper & Row, 1978.

Deal, J., and Deal, L. Efficacy of aphasia rehabilitation: Preliminary results. In R. Brookshire (Ed.), *Clinical aphasiology: Conference proceedings 1978.* Minneapolis: BRK Publishers, 1978.

DeRenzi, E., Pieczuro, A., and Vignolo, L. Oral apraxia and aphasia. *Cortex*, 1966, *2*, 50–73.

DeRenzi, E., and Vignolo, L. The token test: A sensitive test to detect receptive disturbances in aphasics. *Brain*, 1962, *85*, 665–678.

DiSimoni, F., Darley, F., and Aronson, A. Patterns of dysfunction in schizophrenic patients on an aphasia test battery. *J. Speech Hearing Dis.*, 1977, *42*, 498–513.

Dixon, M., and Logue, R. SORRT (Semantic, Oppositional, Rhyming Retrieval Training): A word retrieval program for the anomic patient. Unpublished program 1980.

Duffy, J. Schuell's stimulation approach to rehabilitation. In R. Chapey (Ed.), *Language intervention strategies in adult aphasia.* Baltimore, Md.: Williams & Wilkins, 1981.

Duffy, J., Keith, R., Shane, H., and Podraza, B. Performance of normal (non-brain injured) adults on the Porch index of communicative ability. In R. Brookshire (Ed.), *Clinical aphasiology conference proceedings 1976.* Minneapolis: BRK Publishers, 1976.

Dunham, M., and Newhoff, M. Melodic intonation therapy: Rewriting the song. In R. Brookshire (Ed.), *Clinical aphasiology conference proceedings 1979.* Minneapolis: BRK Publishers, 1979.

Dunn, L. *Peabody picture vocabulary test.* Circle Pines, Minn.: American Guidance Service, 1959.

Eagleson, H., Vaughn, G., and Knudson, A. Hand signals for dysphasia. *Arch. Phys. Med. Rehab.,* 1970, *51,* 111–113.

Edvinsson, L., and Owman, C. Neurovascular aminergic and peptidergic functions in the brain and possible pathophysiological role in cerebral vasospasm. In M. Goldstein, (Ed.), *Advances in neurology 25: Cerebrovascular disorders and stroke.* New York: Raven Press, 1979.

Eisenson, J. Prognostic factors related to language rehabilitation in aphasic patients. *J. Speech Hearing Dis.,* 1949, *14,* 262–264.

Eisenson, J. *Examining for aphasia.* New York: The Psychological Corporation, 1954.

Eisenson, J. Aphasia: A point of view as to the nature of the disorder and factors that determine prognosis for recovery. *Int. J. Neurol.,* 1964, *4,* 287–295.

Eisenson, J. *Adult aphasia: Assessment and treatment.* Englewood Cliffs, N.J.: Prentice-Hall, 1973.

Emerick, L. *Appraisal of language disturbances: Test protocol.* Marquette: Northern Michigan University, 1971.

Ervin-Tripp, S. *Language acquisition and communicative choice.* Stanford, Calif.: Stanford University Press, 1975.

Falek, A., and Britton, S. Phases in coping: The hypothesis and its implications. *Soc. Biol.,* 1974, *21,* 1–7.

Farmer, A., Self-correctional strategies in the conversational speech of aphasic and nonaphasic brain damaged adults. *Cortex,* 1977, *13,* 327–334.

Filby, Y., and Edwards, A. An application of automated-teaching methods to test and teach form discrimination to aphasics. *J. Prog. Instruc.,* 1963, *2,* 25–33.

Flowers, C. How to talk effectively to adult aphasic patients. *J. Minn. Speech Hearing Assoc.,* 1973, *12,* 26–30.

Foley, J. Differential diagnosis of the organic mental disorders in elderly patients. In C. Gaitz (Ed.), *Aging and the brain.* New York: Plenum, 1972.

Fujishima, M., Tanaka, K., Takeya, Y., and Amae, T. Bilateral reduction of hemispheric blood flow in patients with unilateral cerebral infarction. *Stroke,* 1974, *5,* 548–653.

Gardiner, B., and Brookshire, R. Effects of unisensory and multisensory presentation of stimuli upon naming by aphasic patients. *Lang. Speech,* 1972, *15,* 342–357.

Gardner, H., Zurif, E., Berry, T., and Baker, E. Visual communication in aphasia. *Neuropsychologia,* 1976, *14,* 275–292.

Gates, A. *Gates Advanced Primary Reading Test.* New York: Columbia University, Teachers College Press, 1958.

Gates, A., and Bradshaw, J. The role of the cerebral hemispheres in music. *Brain Lang.*, 1977, *4*, 402–431.

Gazzaniga, M., and Hillyard, S. Language and speech capacity of the right hemisphere. *Neuropsychologia*, 1971, *9*, 273–280.

Gazzaniga, M., and Sperry, R. Language after section of the cerebral commissures. *Brain*, 1967, *90*, 131–148.

Geschwind, N. Disconnection syndromes in animals and man. *Brain*, 1965, *88*, 237–294, 585–644.

Geschwind, N. Late changes in the nervous system: An overview. In D. Stein, J. Rosen, and N. Butters (Eds.), *Plasticity and recovery of function in the central nervous system.* New York: Academic Press, 1974.

Gibson, C. Epidemiology and patterns of care of stroke patients. *Arch. Phys. Med. Rehab.*, 1974, *55*, 398–403.

Glass, A., Gazzaniga, M., and Premack, D. Artificial language training in global aphasics. *Neuropsychologia*, 1973, *11*, 95–103.

Gloning, K. Handedness and aphasia. *Neuropsychologia*, 1977, *15*, 355–358.

Godfrey, C. A dysphasia rehabilitation clinic. *Can. Med. Assoc. J.*, 1959, *80*, 616–618.

Godfrey, C., and Douglass, E. The recovery process in aphasia. *Can. Med. Assoc. J.*, 1959, *80*, 618–624.

Goldfarb, A. Memory and aging. In R. Goldman and M. Rockstein (Eds.), *The physiology and pathology of human aging.*

Goldstein, K., *Language and language disturbances.* New York: Grune & Stratton, 1948.

Gonzalez, J., and Aronson, A. Palatal lift prosthesis for treatment of anatomic and neurologic palatopharyngeal insufficiency. *Cleft Pal. J.*, 1970, *7*, 91–104.

Goodglass, H. Studies on the grammar of aphasia. In H. Goodglass and S. Blumstein (Eds.), *Psycholinguistics and aphasia.* Baltimore, Md.: Johns Hopkins University Press, 1973.

Goodglass, H., Barton, M., and Kaplan, E. Sensory modality and object-naming in aphasia. *J. Speech Hearing Res.*, 1968, *11*, 488–496.

Goodglass, H., and Kaplan, E. *The assessment of aphasia and other disorders.* Philadelphia: Lea and Febiger, 1972.

Goodkin, R. Case studies in behavioral research in rehabilitation. *Percept. Motor Skills*, 1966, *23*, 171–182.

Gott, P. Language after dominant hemispherectomy. *J. Neurol., Neurosurg. Psychiat.*, 1973, *36*, 1082–1087.

Green, E., and Boller, F. Features of auditory comprehension in severely impaired aphasics. *Cortex*, 1974, *10*, 133–145.

Hagen, C. Communication abilities in hemiplegia: Effect of speech therapy. *Arch. Phys. Med. Rehab.*, 1973, *54*, 454–463.

Halpern, H., Darley, F., and Brown, J. Differential language and neurologic characteristics in cerebral involvement. *J. Speech Hearing Dis.*, 1973, *38*, 162–173.

Halstead, W., Wepman, J., Reitan, R., and Heimburger, R. *Halstead aphasia test, form M.* Chicago: University of Chicago Industrial Relations Center (undated).

Hardison, D., Marquardt, T., and Peterson, H. Effects of linguistic variables on apraxia of speech. *J. Speech Hearing Res.*, 1977, *13*, 334–343.

Hedrick, D., Christman, M., and Augustine, L. Programming for the antecedent event in therapy. *J. Speech Hearing Dis.*, 1973, *38*, 339–344.

Helm, N. *Melodic intonation therapy: Criteria for candidacy.* Unpublished paper, 1976.

Helm, N. Melodic Intonation Workshop. Corpus Christi, Texas 1977.

Helm, N., and Benson, D. *Visual action therapy for global aphasia.* Paper presented at the Academy of Aphasia, Chicago, 1978.

Helmick, J., Watamori, T., and Palmer, J. Spouses' understanding of the communication disabilities of aphasic patients. *J. Speech Hearing Dis.*, 1976, *41*, 238–243.

Hill, B. *Verbal dyspraxia in clinical practice.* Baltimore, Md.: University Park Press, 1978.

Hoedt-Rasmussen, K., and Skinhoj, E. Transneural depression of the cerebral hemispheric metabolism in man. *Acta Neurol. Scand.*, 1964, *40*, 41–46.

Holland, A. The development and evaluation of programmed instruction techniques for aphasia rehabilitation. USDHEW, Social and Rehabilitation Service: Final Report, Project RD-2361-5-68-C1, 1971.

Holland, A. Case studies in aphasia rehabilitation using programmed instruction. *J. Speech Hearing Dis.*, 1970, *35*, 377–390.

Holland, A. *Aphasics as communicators: A model and its implications.* Paper presented at the American Speech and Hearing Association Convention, Washington, D.C., 1975.

Holland, A. The effectiveness of treatment in aphasia. In R. Brookshire (Ed.), *Clinical aphasiology conference proceedings 1975.* Minneapolis: BRK Publishers, 1975.

Holland, A. Comment on "spouses understanding of the communication disabilities of aphasic patients." *J. Speech Hearing Dis.*, 1977, *42*, 307–308. (a)

Holland, A. Some practical considerations in aphasia rehabilitation. In M. Sullivan & M. Kommers (Eds.), *Rationale for adult aphasia therapy.* Omaha: University of Nebraska Medical Center, 1977. (b)

Holland, A. Functional communication in the treatment of aphasia. In L. Bradford (Ed.), *Communicative disorders: An audio journal for continuing education.* New York: Grune & Stratton, 1978.

Holland, A. Estimates of Aphasic Patients' Communicative Performance in Daily Life. Final Report: NINCDS Grant No. N01-NS-5-2317 1979.

Holland, A. *Communicative abilities of daily living: Test manual.* Baltimore: University Park Press, 1980.

Holland, A., and Harris, A. Aphasia rehabilitation using programmed instruction: An intensive case history. In H. Sloane & B. MacAulay (Eds.), *Operant procedures in remedial speech and language training.* New York: Houghton-Mifflin, 1968.

Holland, A., and Sonderman, J. Effects of a program based on the Token Test for teaching comprehension skills to aphasics. *J. Speech Hearing Res.*, 1974, *17*, 589–598.

Hyman, M. Sociopsychological determinants of patients' performance in stroke rehabilitation. *Arch. Phys. Med. Rehab.*, 1969, *53*, 217–226.

Ingvar, D. Functional landscapes of the dominant hemisphere. *Brain Res.,* 1976, *107,* 181–197.

Jabbari, B., Maulsby, R., Holtzapple, P., and Marshall, N. Prognostic value of EEG in acute vascular aphasia: A long term clinical—EEG study of 53 patients. *Clin. Electroenceph.,* 1979, *10,* 190–197.

Jakobson, R. Toward a linguistic typology of aphasic impairments. In A. DeReuck & M. O'Connor (Eds.), *Disorders of language.* London: Churchill, 1964.

Jenkins, J., Jimenez-Pabon, E., Shaw, R., and Sefer, J. *Schuell's aphasia in adults.* New York: Harper & Row, 1975.

Jerome, E. Decay of heuristic processes in the aged. In C. Tibbits & W. Donahue (Eds.), *Social and psychological aspects of aging.* New York: Columbia University Press, 1963.

Johns, D., and Darley, F. Phonemic variability in apraxia of speech. *J. Speech Hearing Res.,* 1970, *13,* 556–583.

Johns, D., and LaPointe, L. Neurogenic disorders of output processing: Apraxia of speech. In H. Whitaker & H. Whitaker (Eds.), *Studies in neurolinguistics* (Vol. 1). New York: Academic Press, 1976.

Johns, D., and Salyer, K. Surgical and prosthetic management of neurogenic speech disorders. In D. Johns (Ed.), *Clinical management of neurogenic communicative disorders.* Boston: Little, Brown, 1978.

Johnson, J., Somers, R., and Weidner, W. Dichotic ear preference in aphasia. *J. Speech Hearing Res.,* 1977, *20,* 116–129.

Johnson, M. *Recovery from aphasia following traumatic and surgical cortical lesions.* Paper presented at the American Speech and Hearing Association Convention, Washington, D.C., 1975.

Johnt, R., and Goldstein, M. Minor cerebral hemisphere. In W. Friedlander (Ed.), *Advances in neurology* (Vol. 7). New York: Raven Press, 1975.

Jones, L., and Wepman, J. Dimensions of language performance in aphasia. *J. Speech Hearing Res.,* 1961, *4,* 220–232.

Katz, L. Learning in aphasic patients. *J. Consult. Psychol.,* 1958, *22,* 143–146.

Kay, D. Epidemiological aspects of organic brain disease in the aged. In C. Gaitz (Ed.), *Aging and the brain.* New York: Plenum, 1972.

Keenan, J. A method of eliciting naming behavior from aphasic patients. *J. Speech Hearing Dis.,* 1966, *31,* 261–266.

Keenan, J., and Brassell, E. *Aphasia language performance scales (ALPS).* Murfreesboro, Tenn.: Pinnacle Press, 1975.

Keith, R. *Speech and language rehabilitation: A workbook for the neurologically impaired* (Vol. 1). Danville, Ill.: Interstate Printers and Publishers, 1971.

Keith, R. *Speech and language rehabilitation: A workbook for the neurologically impaired* (Vol. 2). Danville, Ill.: Interstate Printers and Publishers, 1977.

Kenin, M., and Swisher, L. A study of recovery in aphasia. *Cortex,* 1972, *8,* 56–68.

Kent, R., and Netsell, R. A case study of an ataxic dysarthric: Cineradiographic and spectrographic observations. *J. Speech Hearing Dis.,* 1975, *40,* 115–134.

Kertesz, A., and McCabe, P. Recovery patterns and prognosis in aphasia. *Brain,* 1977, *100,* 1–18.

Kertesz, A. *Aphasia and Associated Disorders.* New York: Grune and Stratton 1979.

Kertesz, A., and Poole, E. The aphasia quotient: The taxonomic approach to measurement of aphasic disability. *Can. J. Neurol. Sci.,* 1974, *1,* 7–16.

Kimmel, D. *Adulthood and aging: An interdisciplinary developmental view.* New York: John Wiley, 1974.

Kimura, D. The neural basis of language qua gesture. In H. Whitaker & H. Whitaker (Eds.), *Studies in neurolinguistics* (Vol. 2). New York: Academic Press, 1976.

Kinsbourne, M. The minor cerebral hemisphere as a source of aphasic speech. *Arch. Neurol.* 1971, *25,* 302–306.

Kinsbourne, M. Minor hemisphere language and cerebral maturation. In E. Lenneberg & E. Lenneberg (Eds.), *Foundations of language development* (Vol. 2). New York: Academic Press, 1975.

Kohlmeyer, K. Aphasia due to focal disorders of cerebral circulation: Some aspects of localization and of spontaneous recovery. In Y. Lebrun & R. Hoops (Eds.), *Recovery in aphasics.* Amsterdam: Swets and Zeitlinger, 1976.

Krashen, S. Cerebral asymmetry. In H. Whitaker & H. Whitaker (Eds.), *Studies in neurolinguistics* (Vol. 1). New York: Academic Press, 1976.

Kreindler, A., and Fradis, A. *Performances in Aphasia: A Neurodynamical, Diagnostic and Psychological Study.* Paris: Gauthier-Villars 1968.

Kushner, D., and Winitz, H. Extended comprehension practice applied to an aphasic patient. *J. Speech Hearing Dis.,* 1977, *42,* 296–306.

Kushner, D., Hubbard, D., and Knox, A. Effects of punishment on learning by aphasic subjects. *Percept. Motor Skills,* 1973, *36,* 283–289.

Lane, H., and Moore, D. Reconditioning a consonant discrimination in an aphasic: An experimental case history. *J. Speech Hearing Dis.,* 1962, *27,* 232–243.

LaPointe, L. Base-10 programmed stimulation: Task specification, scoring and plotting performance in aphasia therapy. *J. Speech Hearing Dis.,* 1977, *42,* 90–105.

LaPointe, L. Aphasia therapy: Some principles and strategies for treatment. In D. Johns (Ed.), *Clinical management of neurogenic communicative disorders.* Boston: Little, Brown, 1978.

LaPointe, L., and Horner, J. *The reading comprehension battery of aphasia.* Tigard, Ore.: C. C. Publications, 1979.

LaPointe, L., and Johns, D. Some phonemic characteristics in apraxia of speech. *J. Commun. Dis.,* 1975, *8,* 259–269.

Larsen, G. Rehabilitation of dysphagia paralytica. *J. Speech Hearing Dis.,* 1972, *37,* 187–194.

Lasky, E., Weidner, W., and Johnson, J. Influence of linguistic complexity, rate of presentation, and interphrase pause time on auditory-verbal comprehension of adult aphasic patients. *Brain Lang.,* 1976, *3,* 386–395.

Lassen, N., Ingvar, D., and Skinhoj, E. Brain function and blood flow. *Sci. Amer.,* 1978, *239,* 62–71.

LeMay, M., and Geschwind, N. Asymmetries of the human cerebral hemisphere. In A. Caramazza and E. Zurif (Eds.), *Language acquisition and language breakdown.* Baltimore, Md.: Johns Hopkins Press, 1978.

Lenneberg, E. In search of a dynamic theory of aphasia. In E. Lenneberg and E. Lenneberg (eds.), *Foundations of language development, Vol. II.* New York: Academic Press 1975.

Leutenegger, R. *Patient care and rehabilitation of communication-impaired adults.* Springfield, Ill.: Chas. C Thomas, 1975.

Levy, C., and Holland, A. Influence of grammatical complexity and sentence length on comprehension with adult aphasics. In A. Holland, *Psycholinguistics and behavioral variables underlying recovery from aphasia.* Washington, D.C.: Social and Rehabilitation Service, Department of Health, Education, and Welfare, 1971.

Lewis, A. *Mechanisms of neurological disease.* Boston: Little, Brown, 1976.

Liles, B., and Brookshire, R. The effects of pause time on auditory comprehension of aphasic subjects. *J. Comm. Dis.,* 1975, *8,* 221–235.

Lomas, J., and Kertesz, A. Patterns of spontaneous recovery in aphasic groups: A study of adult stroke patients. *Brain Lang.,* 1978, *5,* 388–401.

Long, R. Insights gained through group therapy with multiple sclerosis patients. *J. Nerv. Ment. Dis.,* 1954, *119,* 366.

Longerich, M. *Manual for the aphasia patient.* New York: Macmillan, 1965.

Luria, A. *Restoration of Function After Brain Injury.* New York: Macmillan, 1963.

Luria, A. Factors and forms of aphasia. In A. DeReuck & M. O'Connor (Eds.), *Disorders of language.* London: Churchill, 1964.

Luria, A. *Traumatic aphasia: Its syndrome, psychology and treatment.* The Hague: Mouton, 1970.

Malone, R. Expressed attitudes of families of aphasics. *J. Speech Hearing Dis.,* 1969, *34,* 48–53.

Marks, M., Taylor, M., and Rusk, H. Rehabilitation of the aphasic patient: A summary of three years experience in a rehabilitation setting. *Arch. Phys. Med. Rehab.,* 1957, *38,* 219–226.

Marquardt, T., Rinehart, J., and Peterson, H. Markedness analysis of phonemic substitution errors in apraxia of speech. *J. Comm. Dis.,* 1979, *12,* 312–323.

Marquardt, T., Tonkovich, J., and DeVault, M. Group therapy and stroke club programs for aphasic adults. *J. Tenn. Speech Hearing Assoc.,* 1975, *11,* 2–25.

Marshall, N., and Holtzapple, P. Melodic intonation therapy: Variations on a theme. In R. Brookshire (Ed.), *Clinical aphasiology collected proceedings 1972–1976.* Minneapolis: BRK Publishers, 1978.

Marshall, R. *Clinician-controlled auditory stimulation for aphasic adults.* Tigard, Ore.: C. C. Publications, 1978.

Marshall, R. Word retrieval strategies of aphasic adults in conversational speech. In R. Brookshire (Ed.), *Clinical aphasiology conference proceedings 1975.* Minneapolis: BRK Publishers, 1975.

Marshall, R., and Thistlethwaite, N. *Verbal and nonverbal alerters: Effects on auditory comprehension of aphasic subjects.* Unpublished paper, 1977.

Martin, A. Some objections to the term *apraxia of speech. J. Speech Hearing Dis.,* 1974, *39,* 53–64.

Martin, A. A critical evaluation of therapeutic approaches to aphasia. In R. Brookshire (Ed.), *Clinical aphasiology conference proceedings 1975.* Minneapolis: BRK Publishers, 1975.

Martin, A. Aphasia testing: A second look at the Porch index of communicative ability. *J. Speech Hearing Dis.,* 1977, *42,* 536–546.

Martin, A., and Rigrodsky, S. An investigation of phonological impairment in aphasia, Part 1. *Cortex,* 1974, *10,* 317–327.

Mateer, C., and Kimura, D. Impairment of nonverbal oral movements in aphasia. *Brain Lang.,* 1977, *4,* 262–276.

McDearmon, J., and Potter, R. The use of representational prompts in aphasia therapy. *J. Commun. Dis.,* 1975, *8,* 199–206.

Mchedlishvili, G. Physiological mechanisms controlling cerebral blood flow. *Stroke,* 1980, *11,* 240–248.

McNeil, M., and Prescott, T. *Revised token test.* Baltimore, Md.: University Park Press, 1978.

McNeil, M., Prescott, T., and Chang, E. A measure of PICA ordinality. In R. Brookshire (Ed.), *Clinical aphasiology conference proceedings 1975.* Minneapolis: BRK Publishers, 1975.

McReynolds, L. Contingencies and consequences in speech therapy. *J. Speech Hearing Dis.,* 1970, 12–24.

Meyer, J., Shinohara, Y., Kanda, T., Fukuuchi, Y., Ericsson, A., and Kok, N. Diachisis resulting from acute unilateral cerebral infarction. *Arch. Neurol.,* 1970, *23,* 241–247.

Meyer, J., Welch, K., Okamoto, S., and Shimazu, K. Disordered neurotransmitter function: Demonstration by measurement of Norepinephrine and 5-Hydroxyptamine in CSF patients with recent cerebral infarction. *Brain,* 1974, *97,* 655–664.

Miller, E. *Abnormal ageing.* London: John Wiley, 1977.

Moore, R. Central regeneration and recovery of function: The problem of collateral reinnervation. In D. Stein, J. Rosen, & N. Butters (Eds.), *Plasticity and recovery of function in the central nervous system.* New York: Academic Press, 1974.

Moscovitch, M. On interpreting data regarding the linguistic competence and performance of the right hemisphere: A reply to Selnes. *Brain Lang.,* 1976, *3,* 590–599.

Moscovitch, M. On the representation of language in the right hemisphere of right-handed people. *Brain Lang.,* 1975, *3,* 47–71.

Myers, P., and West, J. The speech pathologist's role with right hemisphere damaged patients. In R. Brookshire (Ed.), *Clinical aphasiology conference proceedings 1978.* Minneapolis: BRK Publishers, 1978.

Naeser, M., Hayward, R., Laughlin, S., and Zatz, L. Quantitative CT scan studies in aphasia: I. Infarct size and CT numbers. *Brain Lang.,* 1981, *12,* 140–164.

Naeser, M., Hayward, R., Laughlin, S., Becker, J., Jernigan, T., and Zatz, L. Quantitative CT scan studies in aphasia: II. Comparison of the right and left hemispheres. *Brain Lang.,* 1981, *12,* 165–189.

National Easter Seal Society for Crippled Children and Adults. *Stroke clubs: How to organize a group program for stroke patients and their families.* Chicago, Ill.: Author, 1972.

Nielsen, J. *Agnosia, apraxia, aphasia.* Los Angeles: Los Angeles Neurological Society, 1936.

Netsell, R. *Kinesiology studies of the dysarthrias.* Madison: University of Wisconsin, 1975.

Netsell, R. Physiologic recordings in the evaluation and rehabilitation of dysarthria. In L. Bradford (Ed.), *Communicative disorders: An audio journal for continuing education.* New York: Grune & Stratton, 1978.

Netsell, R., and Cleeland, C. Modification of lip hypertonia in dysarthria using EMG feedback. *J. Speech Hearing Dis.,* 1973, *38,* 131–140.

Netsell, R., and Daniel, B. Dysarthria in adults: Physiologic approach to rehabilitation. *Arch. Phys. Med. Rehab.,* 1979, *60,* 502–508.

Netsell, R., Daniel, B., and Celesia, G. Acceleration and weakness in Parkinsonian dysarthria. *J. Speech Hearing Dis.,* 1975, *40,* 170–178.

North, A., and Ulatowska, H. *Competence in the independently living elderly: Assessment and correlates.* Unpublished paper, 1979.

Obler, L., Albert, M., Goodglass, H., and Benson, O. Aphasia type and aging. *Brain Lang.,* 1978, *6,* 318–322.

Orgass, B., and Poeck, K. Clinical validation of a new test for aphasia: An experimental study of the token test. *Cortex,* 1966, *2,* 222–243.

Orzeck, A. *Orzeck aphasia evaluation.* Beverly Hills, Calif.: Western Psychological Services, 1964.

Pease, D., and Goodglass, H. The effects of cuing on picture naming in aphasia. *Cortex,* 1978, *14,* 178–189.

Penfield, W., and Roberts, L. *Speech and brain mechanisms.* Princeton, N.J.: Princeton University Press, 1959.

Pettit, J., and Noll, J. Cerebral dominance in aphasia recovery. *Brain Lang.,* 1979, *7,* 191–200.

Porch, B. *Porch index of communicative ability.* Palo Alto, Calif.: Consulting Psychologists Press, 1967, 1971.

Porch, B., Wertz, R., and Collins, M. A statistical procedure for predicting recovery from aphasia. In B. Porch (Ed.), *Proceedings of the conference on clinical aphasiology.* New Orleans, La.: Veterans Administration Hospital, 1974.

Raven, J. *Guide to the standard progressive matrices: Sets A, B, C, D, E.* London: H. K. Lewis, 1960.

Raven, J. *Guide to using the coloured progressive matrices, Sets A, B, Ab.* London: H. K. Lewis, 1963.

Redinger, R., and Dolphin, M. *A new approach to group therapy with aphasic adults.* Paper presented at the American Speech and Hearing Association Convention, New York City, 1970.

Redinger, R., Forster, S., Dolphin, M., Godduhn, J., and Weisinger, J. Group therapy in the rehabilitation of the severely aphasic and hemiplegic in the late stages. *Scand. J. Rehab. Med.,* 1971, *3,* 89–91.

Richardson, A. *Melodic intonation therapy: Theoretical considerations.* Unpublished paper, 1977.

Richardson, A. *Language skills and communication failure in senile dementia.* Doctoral dissertation, University of Texas, 1980.

Rinnert, C., and Whitaker, H. Semantic confusions by aphasic patients. *Cortex,* 1973, *9,* 56–81.

Ritchie, D. *Stroke: A study of recovery.* Garden City, N.Y.: Harper & Row, 1961.

Rochford, G. A study of naming errors in dysphasic and demented patients. *Neuropsychologia,* 1971, *9,* 437–443.

Roland, P. Quantitative assessment of cortical motor dysfunction by measurement of the cerebral blood flow. In R. Fugl-Meyer (Ed.), *Stroke with hemiplegia. Scand. J. Rehab. Med., Suppl. 7,* 1980.

Rosenbek, J. Treating apraxia of speech. In D. Johns (Ed.), *Clinical management of neurogenic communicative disorders.* Boston: Little, Brown, 1978.

Rosenbek, J., Collins, M., and Wertz, R. Intersystemic reorganization for apraxia of speech. In R. Brookshire (Ed.), *Clinical aphasiology collected proceedings 1972–1976.* Minneapolis: BRK Publishers, 1978.

Rosenbek, J., and LaPointe, L. The dysarthrias: Description, diagnosis and treatment. In D. Johns (Ed.), *Clinical management of neurogenic communicative disorders.* Boston: Little, Brown, 1978.

Rosenbek, J., Lemme, M., Ahern, M., Harris, E., and Wertz, R. A treatment for apraxia of speech in adults. *J. Speech Hearing Dis.,* 1973, *38,* 462–472.

Rosenbek, J., and Wertz, R. *Veterans Administration Workshop on Speech Motor Disorders,* Madison, Wis., 1976.

Rosenberg, B. The performance of aphasics on automated visuo-perceptual discrimination, training, and transfer tasks. *J. Speech Hearing Res.,* 1965, *8,* 165–181.

Rosenberg, B., and Edwards, A. The performance of aphasics on three automated perceptual discrimination programs. *J. Speech Hearing Res.,* 1964, *7,* 295–298.

Rosenberg, B., and Edwards, A. An automated multiple response alternative training program for use with aphasics. *J. Speech Hearing Res.,* 1965, *8,* 415–419.

Rosner, B. Recovery of function and localization of function in historical perspective. In D. Stein, J. Rosen, and N. Butters (eds.), *Plasticity of function in the central nervous system.* New York: Academic Press, 1974.

Rubens, A. The role of changes within the central nervous system during recovery from aphasia. In M. Sullivan & M. Kommers (Eds.), *Rationale for adult aphasia therapy.* Omaha: University of Nebraska Medical Center, 1977.

Russell, W. Some anatomical aspects of aphasia. *Lancet,* 1963, *1,* 1173–1177.

Russell, W., and Espir, M. *Traumatic aphasia: A study of aphasia in war wounds of the brain.* London: Oxford University, 1961.

Sands, E., Sarno, M., and Shankweiler, D. Long-term assessment of language function in aphasia due to stroke. *Arch. Phys. Med. Rehab.,* 1969, *50,* 202–207.

Sarno, M. The status of research in recovery from aphasia. In Y. Lebrun & R. Hoops (Eds.), *Recovery in aphasics.* Amsterdam: Swets and Zeitlinger, 1976.

Sarno, M., and Levita, E. Natural course of recovery in severe aphasia. *Arch. Phys. Med. Rehab.*, 1971, *52*, 175–178, 186.

Sarno, M., and Levita, E. Recovery in treated aphasia in the first year post-stroke. *Stroke*, 1979, *10*, 663–670.

Sarno, M., Silverman, M., and Levita, E. Psychosocial factors and recovery in geriatric patients with severe aphasia. *J. Amer. Geriatr. Soc.*, 1970, *18*, 405–409.

Sarno, M., Silverman, M., and Sands, E. Speech therapy and language recovery in severe aphasia. *J. Speech Hearing Res.*, 1970, *13*, 607–623.

Schaie, K., and Strother, C. The effect of time and cohort differences upon age changes in cognitive behavior. *Multivar. Behav. Res.*, 1968, *3*, 259–294. (a)

Schaie, K., and Strother, C. A cross-sequential study of age changes in cognitive behavior. *Psychol. Bull.*, 1968, *70*, 671–680. (b)

Schuell, H. Diagnosis and prognosis in aphasia. *AMA Arch. Neurol. Psychiat.*, 1955, *74*, 308–315.

Schuell, H. A short examination for aphasia. *Neurology (Minneapolis)*, 1957, 625–634.

Schuell, H. *Minnesota test for differential diagnosis of aphasia.* Minneapolis: University of Minnesota Press, 1965.

Schuell, H. A re-evaluation of the short examination for aphasia. *J. Speech Hearing Dis.*, 1966, *31*, 137–147.

Schuell, H., Carroll, V., and Street, B. Clinical treatment of aphasia. *J. Speech Hearing Dis.*, 1955, *20*, 43–53.

Schuell, H., Jenkins, J., and Jimenez-Pabon, E. *Aphasia in adults.* New York: Harper & Row, 1964.

Searle, J. *Speech acts: An essay in the philosophy of language.* Cambridge, England: Cambridge University Press, 1969.

Seron, X., Van der Linden, M., and Van der Kaa-Delvenne. The operant school of aphasia rehabilitation. In Y. Lebrun & R. Hoops (Eds.), *Treatment of aphasia.* Amsterdam: Swets and Zeitlinger, 1978.

Shankweiler, D., and Harris, K. An experimental approach to the problem of articulation in aphasia. *Cortex*, 1966, *2*, 277–292.

Shenkin, H. Bilateral cerebral blood flow: Studies in patients with brain tumor. *Arch. Neurol.*, 1961, *4*, 365–368.

Shewan, C., and Canter, G. Effects of vocabulary, syntax, and sentence length on auditory comprehension in aphasic patients. *Cortex*, 1971, *7*, 209–226.

Shewan, C., and Kertesz, A. Reliability and validity of the Western Aphasia Battery (WAB). *J. Speech Hearing Dis.*, 1980, *45*, 308–324.

Sies, L. (ed.), *Aphasia Theory and Therapy: Selected Lectures and Papers of Hildred Schuell.* Baltimore, Md.: University Park Press, 1974.

Silverman, F. *Communication for the speechless.* Englewood Cliffs, N.J.: Prentice-Hall, 1980.

Skelly, M. *Amer-Ind gestural code based on universal American Indian hand talk.* New York: Elvesier, 1979.

Skelly, M., Schinsky, L., Smith, R., Donaldson, R., and Griffin, J. American Indian sign: A gestural communication system for the speechless. *Arch. Phys. Med. Rehab.*, 1975, *56,* 156–160.

Skelly, M., Schinsky, L., Smith, R., and Fust, R. American Indian Sign (AMERIND) as a facilitator of verbalization for the oral verbal apraxic. *J. Speech Hearing Dis.*, 1974, 39, 445–456.

Sklar, M. *Sklar Aphasia Scale.* Los Angeles: Western Psychological Services, 1966.

Sklar, M. *Sklar aphasia scale.* Beverly Hills, Calif.: Western Psychological Services, 1973.

Smith, A. Speech and other functions after left (dominant) hemispherectomy. *J. Neurol., Neurosurg., Psychiat.,* 1966, *29,* 467–471.

Smith, A. Objective indices of severity of chronic aphasia in stroke patients. *J. Speech Hearing Dis.,* 1971, *36,* 167–207.

Smith, A. *Diagnosis, intelligence and rehabilitation of chronic aphasics.* U.S. Department of Health, Education, and Welfare, Social and Rehabilitation Service: Final Report, Project 14-P55-19815-01, 1972.

Sparks, R. Melodic intonation therapy. In R. Chapey (Ed.), *Language intervention strategies in adult aphasia.* Baltimore, Md.: Williams & Wilkins, 1981.

Sparks, R., Helm, N., and Albert, M. Aphasia rehabilitation resulting from melodic intonation therapy. *Cortex,* 1974, *10,* 303–316.

Sparks, R., and Holland, A. Method: Melodic intonation therapy for aphasia. *J. Speech Hearing Dis.,* 1976, *41,* 287–297.

Spellacy, F., and Spreen, O. A short form of the token test. *Cortex,* 1969, *5,* 390–397.

Spreen, O. Psycholinguistic aspects of aphasia. *J. Speech Hearing Res.,* 1968, *11,* 467–480.

Spreen, O., and Benton, A. *Neurosensory center comprehensive examination for aphasia.* Victoria, B.C.: Neuropsychology Laboratory, University of Victoria, 1969.

Stoicheff, M. Motivating instructions and language performance of dysphasic subjects. *J. Speech Hearing Res.,* 1960, *3,* 75–85.

Strub, R., and Black, F. *The mental status examination in neurology.* Philadelphia: F. A. Davis, 1977.

Stryker, S. *Speech after stroke.* Springfield, Ill.: Chas. C Thomas, 1975.

Subirana, A. The prognosis in aphasia in relation to the factor of cerebral dominance and handedness. *Brain,* 1958, *81,* 415–425.

Swisher, L., and Sarno, M. Token test scores of three matched patient groups: Left brain-damaged with aphasia; right brain-damaged without aphasia; non brain-damaged. *Cortex,* 1969, *5,* 264–273.

Taylor, M. A measurement of functional communication in aphasia. *Archives of physical medicine and rehabilitation,* 1963, *46,* 101–107.

Taylor, M. Language therapy. In H. Burr (Ed.), *The aphasic adult: Evaluation and rehabilitation.* Charlottesville, Va.: Wayside Press, 1964.

Taylor, M., and Marks, M. *Aphasia rehabilitation manual and therapy kit.* New York: McGraw-Hill, 1959.

Templin, M., and Darley, F. *The Templin-Darley Tests of Articulation.* Iowa City: The University of Iowa, 1969.

Terry, R., and Wisniewski, H. Structural aspects of aging of the brain. In C. Eisdorfer & R. Friedel (Eds.), *Cognitive and emotional disturbances in the elderly.* Chicago: Year Book Medical Publishers, 1977.

Tikofsky, R. Two studies of verbal learning by adult aphasics. *Cortex,* 1971, *7,* 106–125.

Tikofsky, R., Kooi, K., and Thomas, M. Electroencephalographic findings and recovery from aphasia. *Neurology (Minneapolis),* 1960, *10,* 154–156.

Tikofsky, R., and Reynolds, G. Further studies of nonverbal learning and aphasia. *J. Speech Hearing Res.,* 1963, *6,* 329–337.

Tomlinson, B., Blessed, G., and Roth, M. Observations on the brains of demented old people. *J. Neurol. Sci.,* 1970, *11,* 205–242.

Tower, D. Effects of ischemia or tissue hypoxia on the neuron. In M. Goldstein, and others (Eds.), *Advances in neurology 25: Cerebrovascular disorders and stroke.* New York: Raven Press, 1979.

Traendly, C. *Aphasia rehabilitation: A speech and language workbook.* Gladstone, Ore.: C.C. Publications, 1977.

Trost, J., and Canter, G. Apraxia of speech in patients with Broca's aphasia: A study of phoneme production accuracy and error patterns. *Brain Lang.,* 1974, *1,* 63–79.

Turnblom, M., and Myers, J. A group discussion program with the families of aphasic patients. *J. Speech Hearing Dis.,* 1952, *17,* 393–396.

Vignolo, L. Evolution of aphasia and language rehabilitation: A retrospective exploratory study. *Cortex,* 1964, *1,* 344–367.

von Monakaw, C. *Die Lokalisation in Grosshirn und der Abbau der Funktion durch kotikale Herde.* Wiesbaden: Bergmann, 1914.

Warren, R. Termination and follow-up: Round table discussion. In R. Brookshire (Ed.), *Clinical aphasiology conference proceedings 1976.* Minneapolis: BRK Publishers, 1976.

Watson, J., and Records, L. The effectiveness of the Porch index of communicative ability as a diagnostic tool in assessing specific behaviors of senile dementia. In R. Brookshire (Ed.), *Clinical aphasiology conference proceedings 1978.* Minneapolis: BRK Publishers, 1978.

Webb, W., and Love, R. *The efficacy of cueing techniques with apraxic-aphasics.* Paper presented to the American Speech and Hearing Association Convention, Las Vegas, Nevada, 1974.

Wechsler, D., and Stone, C. *Wechsler memory scale.* New York: Psychological Corporation, 1948.

Weidner, W., and Lasky, E. The interaction of rate and complexity of stimulus on the performance of adult aphasic subjects. *Brain Lang.,* 1976, *3,* 34–40.

Weigl, E. Neuropsychological experiments on transcoding between spoken and written structures. *Brain Lang.,* 1974, *1,* 227–240.

Weisenburg, T., and McBride, K., *Aphasia: A clinical and psychological study.* New York: Commonwealth Fund, 1935.

Wepman, J. The organization of therapy for aphasia; Inpatient treatment center. *J. Speech Hearing Dis.,* 1947, *12,* 405–409.

Wepman, J. *Recovery from aphasia.* New York: Ronald Press, 1951.

Wepman, J. A conceptual model for the processes involved in recovery from aphasia. *J. Speech Hearing Dis.,* 1953, *18,* 4–13.

Wepman, J. The relationship between self-correction and recovery from aphasia. *J. Speech Hearing Dis.,* 1958, *23,* 302–305.

Wepman, J., and Jones, L. *The Language Modalities Test for Aphasia.* Chicago: Education-Industry Service, 1961.

Wertz, R. Neuropathologies of speech and language: An introduction to patient management. In D. Johns (Ed.), *Clinical management of neurogenic communication disorders.* Boston: Little, Brown, 1978.

Wertz, R., Brookshire, R., Holtzapple, M., Hubbard, D., Porch, B., & West, J. Veterans Administration cooperative study on the effects of speech and language therapy on recovery from aphasia. In B. Porch (Ed.), *Proceedings of the conference on clinical aphasiology.* New Orleans, La.: 1974.

Wertz, R., Collins, M., Weiss, D., Brookshire, R., Friden, T., Kurtzke, J., and Pierce, J. *Veterans Administration cooperative study of aphasia: Preliminary report on a comparison of individual and group treatment.* Paper presented to the American Association for the Advancement of Science, Washington, D.C., 1978.

Wertz, R., Rosenbek, J., and Deal, J. A review of 228 cases of apraxia of speech: Classification, etiology, and localization. Paper presented at American Speech and Hearing Association Convention, New York 1970.

West, J. Auditory comprehension in aphasic adults: Improvement through training. *Arch. Phys. Med. Rehab.,* 1973, *54,* 78–86.

West, J. The concept of diaschisis: A reply to Markowitsch and Pritzel. *Behav. Biol.,* 1978, *22,* 413–416.

Whitaker, H. A case of the isolation of the language function. In H. Whitaker & H. Whitaker (Eds.), *Studies in neurolinguistics,* (Vol. 2). New York: Academic Press, 1976.

Wiersma, W., and Klausmier, H. The effect of age upon speed of concept attainment. *J. Geront.,* 1965, *20,* 398–400.

Wilcox, M., and Davis, G. Speech act analysis of aphasic communication in individual and group settings. In R. Brookshire (Ed.), *Clinical aphasiology conference proceedings 1977.* Minneapolis: BRK Publishers, 1977.

Wilcox, M., and Davis, G. *Promoting aphasics' communicative effectiveness* (PACE). Memphis, Tenn.: Memphis State University, 1978.

Wilcox, M., Davis, G., and Leonard, L. Aphasics' comprehension of contextually conveyed meaning. *Brain Lang.,* 1978, *6,* 362–377.

Yarnell, P., Monroe, P., and Sobel, L. Aphasia outcome in stroke: A clinico neuroradiological correlation. *Stroke,* 1976, *7,* 516–522.

Yorkston, K., and Beukelman, D. An analysis of connected speech samples of aphasic and normal speakers. *J. Speech Hearing Dis.,* 1980, *45,* 27–36.

Yorkston, K., Marshall, R., and Butler, M. Imposed delay of response: Effects on aphasics auditory comprehension of visually and non-visually cued material. *Percep. Motor Skills,* 1977, *44,* 647–655.

Young, M. Problem-solving performance in two age groups. *J. Geront.,* 1966, *21,* 505–509.

Zaidel, E. Unilateral auditory language comprehension on the token test following cerebral commissurotomy and hemispherectomy. *Neuropsychologia,* 1977, *15,* 1–15.